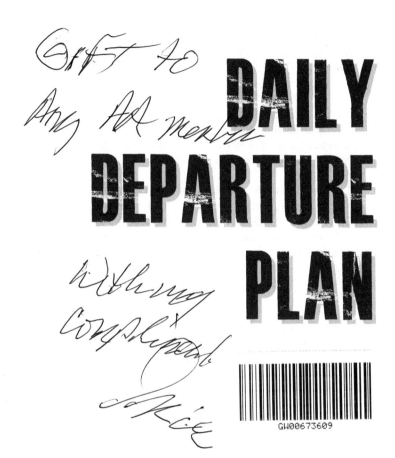

DAILY DEPARTURE PLAN

GW00673609

by Mike C.

MYSTIC SUNSET
PUBLISHING

JACKSONVILLE, FL

Daily Departure Plan
A Daily Meditation in Memoir For Those in Recovery
Copyright ©2021 by Mike C.

This meditation in memoir is a collection of the author's communications with his sponsees in AA. They include interactions with family and friends and life events. Some events have been shifted on the timeline for flow purposes only. Some names and identifying details have been changed to protect the privacy of others.

Edited by Lynn Skapyak Harlin
Layout and Design by Richard Levine
Cover Design by Shannon Cavanaugh
Cover Photo by James Fox

The information contained in this book is the author's personal experience and should not be considered a substitute for the advice of a qualified medical professional specializing in addiction disorders.

ISBN 979-8-9852436-0-4

MYSTIC SUNSET
PUBLISHING

Printed in the United States of America

I dedicate this book to my son, Michael who departed at age 61, during the writing of this book. He left us much too early, September 27, 2020 on the birthday of his brother who also departed even earlier at age 56. The loss of my two sons inspired me not only to have a *Daily Flight Plan* but also have a *Daily Departure Plan*. I continue to write meditations for my children and grandchildren as a living amends.

ACKNOWLEDGMENTS

Heartfelt gratitude goes out to the entire fellowship of Alcoholics Anonymous. A special thanks to my home group of the last 16 years, Good Morning Pattaya. My first home group, the Wailana Group in Honolulu, Hawaii gave me a great start for 11 years. AA saved my life so that I may be of service to my still suffering alcoholic brothers and sisters. I received unconditional love from the very first day of sobriety and hopefully this book will pass on that love to others which was freely given to me.

My Jacksonville Team, consisting of my two daughters, Shannon and Diane doing editing, artwork and the logistics of getting this printed. It was a team love project and I am truly blessed to have such a wonderful family. *Daily Flight Plan* has enjoyed a long run due to diligent efforts the JAX Team.

Lynn Skapyak Harlin, my amazing editor, worked tirelessly for a year to assist me complete this project. Lynn has great hopes I will be a writer someday.

INTRODUCTION

The author of these daily messages for each day of the year is Mike C. As an active member of Alcoholics Anonymous he got sober in Hawaii with a sobriety date of April 21, 1994. After 11 years in the program he moved to Thailand and these short messages began as a method for Mike to keep in touch with men he sponsored in recovery. Over the years he has added sponsees from over 10 different locations all over the map. The writings offered here are selected from 20 years of carrying the message of AA.

Mike is a retired military officer and a combat pilot with 29 years of service. In addition to being an alcoholic he suffers from PTSD from his years in Vietnam, Laos, Thailand and Afghanistan. He shares his experience, strength and hope to include the loss of two sons, one to ALS disease in 2017, and another son in 2020 from alcoholism.

Mike stresses to the people he sponsors: prayer, readings and meditation upon awakening every morning. The use of a gratitude list is repeated in the pages that follow. The idea of this book is to read one page, every day, over a cup of coffee. Here is a list of the books Mike reads every single morning:

Alcoholics Anonymous (4th Edition). Commonly referred to as *The Big Book*.

Daily Reflections. Also an AA publication.

Body Mind and Spirit. A Hazelden Publication.

Twenty-Four Hours A Day. A Hazelden Publication.

Around the Year by Emmet Fox. A Harper One Publication.

A New Day. A Bantam Book.

The Twelve Step Prayer Book. A Hazelden Publication.

Here are the 12 Steps of Alcoholics Anonymous that are suggested as a program of recovery:

Step 1: We admitted we were powerless over alcohol—that our lives had become unmanageable.

Step 2: Came to believe that a Power greater than ourselves could restore us to sanity.

Step 3: Made a decision to turn our will and our lives over to the care of God as we understood Him.

Step 4: Made a searching and fearless moral inventory of ourselves.

Step 5: Admitted to God, to ourselves, and to another human being the exact nature of our wrongs.

Step 6: Were entirely ready to have God remove all these defects of character.

Step 7: Humbly asked Him to remove our shortcomings.

Step 8: Made a list of all persons we had harmed and became willing to make amends to them all.

Step 9: Made direct amends to such people wherever possible, except when to do so would injure them or others.

Step 10: Continued to take personal inventory and when we were wrong promptly admitted it.

Step 11: Sought through prayer and meditation to improve our conscious contact with God, as we understood Him, praying only for knowledge of His will for us and the power to carry that out.

Step 12: Having had a spiritual awakening as the result of these Steps, we tried to carry this message to alcoholics, and to practice these principles in all our affairs.

DAILY MEDITATIONS

January 1

PATH OF LOVE

There are many paths to the summit where all paths meet. The one open to all is the path of love. The other two paths are the path of knowledge and the path of action. The discussion today is the love path because I am a love-bug. I never get tired speaking about love. One of my daily prayers says, "Speak your love. Speak it again." My prayers emphasize love, my day starts and ends with love. The path of love is where I want to be. To me, gratitude, love, forgiveness, joy, happiness is one melody of harmony. I am convinced God Is Love. God loves me and all my brothers and sisters equally.

Love removes my fears because love is also faith. True attainment of my goal of a spiritual awakening is through the yoga of Love. Yoga means union and our union with God makes our goals attainable. In order to grow on the love path, I must also love every human being. They are my brothers and sisters. This becomes difficult if we have an enemies list, resentments and prejudice. There is no act God does not forgive, how dare I hold back my forgiveness to anyone, no matter what they have done. I can't help someone unless they are attracted to me in some way. Love fills in all the blanks missing in life.

Before I decided to pick this path of love, I had no concept of a loving Higher Power. My mind was slammed shut. The word God meant judgment and condemnation. How wrong can one person be? Love is the answer.

OWNERSHIP

What do you own? A house, a car, land and a bank account. You may be a steward of some stuff temporarily but houses need repair, a car will end up in the junk yard sooner or later. Land belongs to Mother Earth. You may be privileged to occupy some for a short time. The only thing I own is my thoughts, character, attitude and actions. I have made a point of giving up ownership of "stuff". My feelings I do own. If I am angry, I need to own it and only I can stop the emotion before it leads to an action I will surely regret. On the positive side I own my happiness. It does not depend on somebody else and it is not attached to material well-being.

On a ranch the owner of all the livestock puts a brand on his animals to insure he gets back his strays. We have a circle with a triangle on signs to tell us what is AA or where a meeting might be. There is no ownership in AA. It is not a company or corporation. When a visitor comes into our meeting room, he or she sees a clean room with lights on, books out, coffee pot on, the 12 Steps on the wall and friendly members. No owners. My actions have my "brand" on it for good or bad. My attitude I do own.

When the last curtain comes down, I would like to be remembered by the people I have helped. Whatever I had temporary stewardship over in life is of no consequence.

YOUR BUTTONS

So much of my early life was full of hurt feelings. It seemed like the whole world made me feel inferior. Everything was personal and hurtful. Dreams of being a writer were smashed by teachers insulting my writing. "You are foggier than London." Plus, a lousy C grade when all my other subjects were A's. As a result, I gave up my dream. When I finally started a life of recovery, I heard concepts new to me. "Nobody can make you feel bad without your permission." And "What other people think of me is none of my business." People pleasing was one of my horrible character defects. My buttons were open to be pushed. Some folks knew just how to push my buttons.

Still to this day I am triggered by certain events or verbal button pushing. The difference, however, is I am aware of my sensitivities and put myself on hold before I act or open my mouth. Someone talking down to me in a condescending way is one example. Since I don't do it, I don't appreciate being addressed as a child. Today I don't react when it happens even though I still don't like it. Another example is a male abusing a female verbally or physically. My gut reaction is to intervene but not a good idea in some cases. Caution required.

My good friend Rick, who has long passed away, gave me this thought I carry with me. "Mike, if somebody pushes your buttons, they are your buttons. You installed them so you can remove them."

FREE EDUCATION

In school and college, I learned calculus, cost accounting, aerodynamics but never how to live my life. It wasn't until I made my way into recovery, the education I really needed and could use, began. The best part is this education is free. No entry tests required just be sober and show up for class also known as a meeting. There are many classes near you. The teachers are hardened experienced folks who have been in the testing lab for decades ready to share their knowledge free of charge. These teachers will tell you what worked for them and what did not. Some will not apply so it is a good idea to listen carefully to pick out what fits your situation.

Some of the teachers in the meetings relate horror stories from real life events you can avoid by taking the lesson to heart and not trying the same thing. In meetings I often heard the drug related stories over the years. In my case, drugs were never part of my story. I know from my education in meetings to be careful of pain killers when offered by the doctor. Many of my friends have lost it all to one pill too many. I have witnessed wet brain in living color and maybe one more martini there go I. Never did I get a course in Relationships 101 until I attended class regularly. I go to meetings to find out what happens to people who quit going to meetings.

The gems learned in meetings are more valuable than gold. These jewels are available to all but you need to be there since we don't make recordings or do videos. The education is ongoing for the rest of your life. Best deal on the planet.

January 5

HOW TO WIN AN ARGUMENT

Argument was the order of the day around my house when I was growing up. My mother had an overwhelming stream of verbiage directed at me so I caved in rather than engage in dialogue. I never was good at arguing but I kept trying and losing face constantly. I have found most alcoholics suffer from the same weakness. Once I am angry, reason evaporates and I become stupid. When I do come to my senses, I become brilliant again after the battle is over and my adversary is sound asleep. Some folks love to argue because they are good at it. I have learned to stay away from these types and refuse to join the fight.

I never could master the art of argument without anger. The cool one seems to get the upper hand and I am not a "cool" one. If I know I am right I can keep it to myself and let the other guy think he is right. Only God knows what is right for sure. One of my prayers says, "Let me not rejoice in who is right but in what is right." The fallout from argument is worse than the value of the point to be made. Relationships get damaged and a negative cloud becomes the order of the day. Anger in any form is a threat to my positive way of thinking. I can't afford the loss of serenity. Resentments galore, hurt feelings and amends to be made, no thank you.

How do you win an argument? Give it to your Higher Power. Let the wrong party get it set straight from God. Leave yourself out of the equation. Every argument I walk away from makes me a winner.

January 6

BRIGHT SPOTS

It is hard to remember a bright spot when I was drinking since there were not many. If somebody gave me a bottle of whiskey as a gift it would be a bright spot. A pay raise might do it. Only if I got something would I say something is a bright spot. Today my entire thought process has reversed. To see my friends succeed is brighter than any success of mine. To witness a broken-down drunk, get sober and become a useful member of society is a bright spot not to be missed. Today my bright spots are not about me but focus on my brothers and sisters. Their love and friendship bring me joy to light up my life.

If I can help someone come out of depression and smile again, I am rewarded. What a difference from the days when I was not capable of helping anyone. Selfishness has no bright spots. Whatever you get is never enough. Giving of yourself brings a brightness with a multiplier effect. Every day I communicate with a host of friends who love me. Their love fires up my engine and I think of ways to love them back. My day is full of bright spots as I go about giving instead of taking. The loving companionship of others feeds my soul with laughter and happiness.

From the old days of isolation to today, my arms are open to the love of others. I never thought I deserved the time and attention of others. Now it is the air I breathe.

January 7

I KNOW

"Each man can interpret another's experience only by his own," quote from Henry David Thoreau. The sweetest words I heard at my first AA meeting was, "I know." I was pouring out my woes and problems and several people said, "I know." As I looked into their eyes, I could see they, in fact, did know. The experience of alcoholics is remarkably similar. It was great comfort to me when I started my road to recovery to be understood. I thought I was unique. What a joke. I fit right in from day one. There was no doubt I belonged in AA. I was years late for my first meeting. The experience of those who went before me took me out of the fog.

When I started sponsoring other alcoholics, it was my turn to say, "I know." My experience, strength and hope put me on level ground with the guys I tried to help. Whatever pain they shared with me I could offer empathetic words with sincerity. We became brothers in suffering but also in a spiritual awakening. When my son passed away another member lost his son four days before. It cut my grief in half instantly. Every meeting I attend is rich in experience. I learn what works and what doesn't work. Whatever happens to me, somebody in the fellowship will say, "I know."

One alcoholic helping another is the heart and soul of Alcoholics Anonymous. It takes one to know one.

RIGHT OR LEFT?

My life has been full of turning points. Some were turn right is life and turn left is death. Some were out of my control. Such as being assigned to Maine instead of Arizona because the guy making assignments was selling locations and I was not offered the deal. Some were pure luck. I picked mission A with no problems and mission B ended up being shot down. My most important turning point was to put down the drink and enter the road to recovery. Today I enjoy turning points because my Higher Power is part of the equation. I have faith every turning point is the right one.

As I get older, I have medical turning points which require accepting new limitations and adjustments of my life style. Hopefully, these opportunities will extend my life a few more days. On the good side, I have spiritual turning points taking me to higher awakening plateaus and knowledge. These are more up than right or left as my spirit is lifted to even more happiness. Sometimes I feel like levitating and flying without wings. All the jogs and twists of life have turned out just like God intended. They all brought me to this exact spot, on planet Earth, in my present condition and circumstances. I could not have designed a better plan.

If I do the "next right thing" enough times in a row I am confident I am in the correct zone. Today I seek help when faced with a decision. My Higher Power gives me bursts of inspiration which guide my intuition.

SELECT A MEMORY

"I have more memories than if I were a thousand years old," quote from Charles Baudelaire. One of my blessings is a good memory. I can remember my drill instructors name from sixty years back. The day my father came home from WWII in 1945 happened yesterday in my memory. At 80 years old my memory tape room has enough memory stored to fill a library. How I use this memory is part of my spiritual path. It could be a curse if I am not careful. It is a blessing when I can pull out a memory to help another person. Just like attitude, I can control my memories and use them properly. In my morning meditation memories flood my consciousness, both good and bad.

Right now, I am writing stories of my past life to honor a promise to my children. I want my writing to be the truth and not create a fractured fairy tale. The truth is I was selfish and egotistical for a large chunk of my life. It is painful to bring these memories back to life after I buried them during recovery. The process has made me grateful my life has a spiritual center. I am blessed to still be alive to complete the task. One memory I keep green in my mind is my bottom in 1993. I can recall the sickness, demoralization, and despair as if it were an hour ago. I am in charge of picking the memory tapes from storage. I pick "bottom" every day.

My Higher Power helps me pick the memories which might help someone. He also brings back sweet memories such as the birth of my children. I can focus on the joy instead of the pain.

January 10

FAILURE IS SUCCESS

When I pray, I know it will be successful. I might not see immediate results and think my prayers failed. My spiritual teachers caution me not to get ahead of God. Maybe my prayer will be answered years down the road in God's time, not mine. I can see throughout my life what appeared to be a failure was success in disguise. God's plan reveals itself if you remain patient and have faith. Becoming a hopeless drunk seems like a failure. Yet it led me to a new life of joy and happiness. If I wasn't a drunk first, I may never have found the wonderful life I have today.

Success or failure is a judgment call. A lot depends on your attitude, positive or negative. If you label something a failure and stop taking action you will be correct. It is a failure. I am reminded of the story of Colonel Sanders and his recipe for fried chicken. He went to a hundred different companies who labeled his idea a failure. He kept the faith and tried one more source. The result is one of the largest fast-food franchises on the planet. KFC is a billion-dollar company with outlets in 150 countries.

I could have been a complete failure if I didn't keep my faith and follow my heart. My sobriety is a daily success.

OUR INNERMOST SELVES

Admitting I was an alcoholic happened when I was 25 years old but it was OK with me. I could not see any consequences. There were three of us in the same class at the bar at 11 p.m. often and one guy was worried about becoming an alcoholic. For me, no worries, it was part of the job in my mind. "Hey guys we are functional, no hangovers and still perform well on the job. So what?" It took years for bad stuff to happen and by then my goose was cooked. More About Alcoholism page 30 in the Big Book says, "We learned that we had to fully concede to our innermost selves that we were alcoholics." Never once did I search my inner self. Way too scary to look.

Thirty years after the first admission I was alcoholic, I did both parts of the first step. Today I am happy to be an alcoholic because I know what I am 100%. Before I did a real Step One, I did not know who I was. There was the person I wanted to be and the person I pretended to be but neither was reality. The recovery process brought me to ground zero of the real me. The admission was a spiritual awakening and a great starting point to begin a new and different life. Inside the innermost self I found God who was there all the time patiently waiting for me to wake up.

When I learned to examine my inner self there was much to find besides the fact, I was an alcoholic. There were parts of who I really was hidden from my forward view. Today the real me is out in the open.

TWELVE STEP ADVENTURE

A Twelve Step call is always an adventure. You never know what to expect. You can be received by the person needing help with open arms. Then again, you might get thrown out with foul language and physical threats. Quite often the call for help comes from the spouse or a friend who has no idea what to do. In frustration and desperation, the family member calls the AA hotline. I recommend caution if the call is not from the drunk himself. Also, you should have at least two sober alcoholics to make the visit. Once in the presence of the still suffering person, never talk down to him or her. Establish your alcoholism, be friendly and humble.

The first few moments of a Twelve Step call can set the tone for good results. If the person is willing to talk, you are off to a good start. In the process of conversation, if the person admits to having a drinking problem you are on level ground. Now you can establish all of us present have a drinking problem. The two of us making the visit were at one time as bad off as the person needing help but now, we have been sober a while. The AA tag team can then explain how we stay sober. A helping hand is out and support is readily available. If possible, getting the person to his or her first meeting right after the visit is recommended. If all goes well the AA team can cart off the bottle of vodka on the table.

A Twelve Step call is always successful to the AA members participating. You are reaching out. Leave the results up to God. The seed has been planted.

January 13

ENTHUSIASM

"Nothing great was ever achieved without enthusiasm," quote from Ralph Waldo Emerson. Having enthusiasm for living shows the world you have fire in the furnace. Enthusiasm comes from a positive attitude and faith. Good things will happen. Enthusiasm breathes hope into our resolve to live a happy sober lifestyle. There is a spirit of fun added into the formula of enthusiasm. Being upbeat has a ripple effect on others and can be contagious. I start each day with great enthusiasm. Even though I say the same prayers every morning I put new zip into my attitude and focus on some phrases to keep my prayers fresh. Today I focused on this line: "To be just as enthusiastic about the success of others as I am about my own."

One of my good friends with 40 plus years of sobriety shares the enthusiasm of a kid with a new toy. Full of life, hope, and fun. He inspires all who listen to his sharing. A super example for me to follow always looking for new ways to show my deep enthusiasm. When my heart is full of gratitude it shows on my face and hopefully in my speech. Love is in every fiber of my existence. I want to project all this joy outward to help others.

Enthusiasm is an action word. It is the fruit of positive action. As I get older I find the simple things in life light my fire. To witness spiritual progress is thrilling.

POISON TONGUE

Your tongue can be as deadly as a snake bite. Your venom is poison not only to your victim but to you as well. It seems to be human nature to gossip about people who are not present to defend themselves. My practice was to stay at the bar until everyone was gone so nobody could gossip about me. I guess some folks feel superior in some way by running someone else down and doing the inventory of others. In AA we would like to think our program teaches us "love and tolerance". Let a physical confrontation happen in the rooms and it will travel across the globe faster than electricity. The AA tongues wag with the best of them.

Whatever I don't like about someone is best kept to myself. As soon as I verbalize to someone else, I am spreading poison. It is not my job to correct my fellows or judge them lest I be judged. Being critical is a negative endeavor and it is none of my business anyway. Usually, a joke is at someone's expense. I try to keep my joking about my own pratfalls. I have to remember what Thumper taught me 70 years ago in Bambi a Walt Disney movie, "If you can't say nothing nice about somebody don't say nothing at all." You need to be careful with alcoholics, they are sensitive.

Once you say something it is in stone for all time. You cannot take it back. Things I have said decades ago still bite me. Better to pause and consider your comments. Maybe silence is the best route to peace and good will.

PRAYER IS ALWAYS THE ANSWER

My spiritual adviser has taught me prayer should never be a chore or a task. Prayer is not mental drudgery. It is a loving expression to your friend, God. A short, from the heart prayer is just as effective as an epistle. Actually, you need not think too much about method or style of prayer because it is your conversation with your Higher Power. I look forward to my prayer time and enjoy the process. It is a joyful time of my day, refreshing and energy producing. Prayer is always the answer to whatever problem I might be wrestling with. I don't pray because I must. I pray because I want to. I am limited but God has no limits. We are a team.

Prayer without faith does not work. If I pray for bread and don't bring a basket, a lack of faith is clear. First the request goes to your Higher Power then action on your part such as taking practical steps toward a solution. Your prayers will be answered. The answer may not come as you expect or when you expect it. When I was in deep trouble with a real possibility of losing my life, I prayed. Even though I was a dead man walking I kept taking action. I am still here is my best evidence. I pray quietly, relax and leave the rest up to my Higher Power. I have never been disappointed.

In my morning mediation I say eight prayers without fail. They inspire me, give gratitude to my Higher Power who made this great life possible and spared me from death's door many times over.

January 16

NO HEROES HERE

Mickey Mantel, the Yankee baseball player, was my first hero. Then I joined the military where heroes are treated like saints. Air Force heroes, Chuck Yeager and Robin Olds were put up on a pedestal for junior bird-men like me to honor. When I became a combat pilot, I received several awards labeling me a hero. I knew better and did not like being called a hero. My awards came from doing my job as I was trained for the most part. Some high awards were from circumstances of survival. Just because I made it out alive does not make me a hero. I'm no hero. I'm a drunk. That's the truth.

The most meaningful organization I ever joined was the fellowship of AA. No heroes in AA. In fact, the Traditions of AA caution against leaders and personalities. Our literature states it is unfair to a fellowship member to treat them as a hero. Each one of us is one drink away from going back to the bottom as a drunk. No member is special or a poster child for the program. There is no CEO or president. No matter how charismatic or length of sobriety a member might have, he or she remains anonymous. The man with fifty years of continuous sobriety is equal to the man who just walked in the door. All of us have only 24 hours of sobriety, the record amount.

Our founders knew the dangers of the limelight. If a hero falls it reflects on the entire program. Sobriety is my daily reward. I don't need a medal.

STAKE YOUR CLAIM

In the Old West during the Gold Rush folks from the East traveled West to "stake their claim". You could post your spot in the ground as your own in the dream of finding gold and prosperity. In recovery we can do the same thing. We can seek a home group we can call "our" home group. Of course, to claim it you need to attend meetings regularly. Then offer yourself in service to this particular group as part of the deal. As an active member you greet new arrivals and guests as a "homie". Once you have roots by staking your claim you are available to help others and enjoy the fruits of the best fellowship on earth.

A key "stake your claim" part of recovery is to have a personal spot for your daily prayer and meditation. I have my corner on the kitchen table. It is my temple, my church, and secret meeting place with my Higher Power with no distractions. Quieting the mind is a must. The first hour of the day is the most important part of my recovery even before I head out to my home group. My sobriety is the most precious stake of my existence. My prayer is asking God to remove those character defects standing in the way of helping others.

We all have a tool kit to work our claim. Plenty of literature, meetings of all sorts, a telephone, and a computer. Gold is in my claim and I will mine it for the rest of my life.

TEACHERS AND PREACHERS

Who's the boss? My question for my first AA meeting. Only trusted servants I was told. Impossible I thought, but after I learned how this fellowship operates, I love it. I don't need to be a boss anymore and Lord knows I hated bosses. No rank structure in AA which is perfect for us. Then I heard AA is not a religion, no preachers. Good to hear in principle even if we do hear some preaching in meetings. I loved being a teacher in my professional life but I had to give up the podium for a seat in the group. Nobody is better than anybody else no matter how much sobriety or how educated a person might be. Being smart will not keep you sober I have found.

What we have is anarchy. Most people think that means chaos but it really means total freedom of the individual. No government. Yes, we have our Traditions but even they are "suggested". The Steps and Traditions don't include the words don't or can't. The Steps tell me what to do and the not part I can figure out for myself. Nowhere do I see "don't drink" but it becomes obvious. The only inventory I am responsible for is my own and teaching others is not my job. I can say what worked for me in my experience.

Bottom line, we will hear bullies, preachers, and teachers. Some folks need to vent their anger at meetings which makes me grateful for my serenity. A lot of what is said in meetings I let blow in the wind but I save the gems.

January 19

NIP IT IN THE BUD

"Meet the first beginning; look to the budding mischief before it has time to ripen to maturity," quote from William Shakespeare. My sister often signs off on her messages with, "I need to go pull out some weeds before they become trees." Same is true for the weeds in your life. A tiny problem can grow into major catastrophe if you don't nip it in the bud. I heard a noise when I took a shower like a bee buzzing. I wrote it off as nature outside my house. The buzzing sound became louder over time until it gave me a headache. A city of termites had invaded the wall behind my shower and a section of my house had to be replaced and the house tented.

I try to keep my relationships in good repair. A small slight can eventually ripen into a resentment. Most of my communication is by message since I live in Thailand. The disadvantage of words on a screen is they lack tone of voice and other body language. I may think I am being funny but the recipient of my message might take offense. Once I detect a misunderstanding in the bud, I nip it. Taking care of your body when you become a dinosaur is a challenge. A small black spot on your skin can kill you if you ignore it. A tiny pain in a tooth can lead to a wide gap in your smile.

Procrastination and fear can cause us to skip over small "weeds" in our life. If you address problems before they take root it will keep your garden clean. Get'em when they are young.

RISK TAKING

Fear of looking stupid never stopped me from taking risks. Growing up I was a bit of a dare devil to get attention and doing dangerous risky stuff became part of my character. The military life was perfect for me. The higher the risk the better the payoff. Once I joined the pilot community, I could have been a transport pilot, safe with little risk. Transport pilots were referred to as trash haulers. The need for a combat pilot assignment was essential to advancement. Screw the risk. Once inside the combat community they had special risky missions for idiots like me. Somehow God saved me so I could write to you guys about risk taking. Risking your life for recognition is insane.

An examination of motive is required for risk taking. Consulting your Higher Power and your sponsor is probably a good idea. In my case I took risks to push myself up the ranks and gain recognition. It worked but the motive was corrupt thus not really success. Think about all the risks of driving drunk. Some of us did it again and again until we hit something or got caught. Thank God those kinds of risks are history. No more life and death risks. Of course, just being on the roadway is a risk but now I buckle up. My children and grand kids love me and need me alive.

Risk taking is a balance between faith and fear. Hopefully we indulge in reasonable risks to achieve new horizons. You won't read about me skydiving at 80.

THE TAIL IS WAGGING THE DOG

Dogs are very honest. They look you straight in the eye. If their tail is wagging you have passed the friend or foe test. People on the other hand lie, "good to see you" when they are thinking the opposite. Lucky human beings don't have a tail or else our tails would tell the truth. We let anger and resentments wag us. We can change our attitude and stop letting other people wag us to death. Some of us never learn not to let the events of the world ruin our emotional temperature. I follow the example of the dogs. Look the world in the eye.

We tend to let temporary things wag us around. Being defeated is temporary but giving up is permanent. Committing suicide is a permanent solution to a temporary problem but we see fellow members choose death as an option. The control of our mental faculties is all important to stop the tail wagging. Prayer is the best tool for help on any problem. God could and would if sought yet we don't seek Him when we need to. Why in the world do we try to solve situations when we are part of the problem instead of looking outside ourselves? The courage to continue is what counts. Tenacity.

Mistakes made me what I am today. I have learned so much from temporary failure. I have had to put my tail between my legs many times but today life doesn't wag me to death.

January 22

THE QUIET LIFE

"A happy life must be to a great extent a quiet life, for it is only in an atmosphere of quiet that true joy can live," quote from Bertrand Russell. In my bar hopping days I would peek into a bar and if it was too quiet, I moved on. I craved noisy places. I had a bumper sticker, "Jet noise, the Sound of Freedom." What a crock. Jet noise is what destroyed my hearing. I enjoyed chaos in my drinking career. Noise was part of the chaos. Now I have gone the other way and embrace peace and quiet. I can't take a noisy gathering anymore. When I work with another alcoholic, I meet them in the quietest coffee shop or restaurant.

My first hour of every day is totally noiseless. Prayer and meditation work best for me when it is quiet. I can concentrate and listen for messages from my Higher Power. God has never shouted at me. I need to listen to my heart thus I need quiet to pick up the tiny voice within. I welcome quiet, seek it and am grateful for the lack of turmoil in my daily affairs. I keep my mouth quiet also. I don't need to hear the sound of my voice or spend time in meaningless conversation. When I share in an AA meeting, I am brief. The only way I can write is to quiet my mind and shut out any static.

Today I live a quiet life. Serenity and noise just don't mix well. I don't need the quick pace of excitement to enjoy life.

OUR OWN BED OF NAILS

Many years ago, I witnessed a group of men walking the streets of Tehran beating themselves with chains to the point of blood flowing down their backs. Pretty extreme in our culture but alcoholics are past masters at self-flagellation verbally and mentally. Deep depression from low self-esteem was common in most of the guys I sponsored. Encouragement and positive reinforcement worked well in those cases. I blamed bad luck and other people for my problems. When my inventory was finished it was clear I needed to own my troubles and claim my character defects. Yes, I designed my own private bed of nails.

When you need a friend the most, why not look in the mirror? Self-love may take some time after years of low esteem. Hitting bottom usually is a collection of defeats not just one event. It may take a ton of victories to begin to befriend yourself. Every day without drinking is a victory. Repairing your body from years of neglect is another victory. Experiencing the spiritual awakening the program promises is a huge plateau to reach. God loves you, all the members of your group love you, so what are you waiting for? Your own mental attitude can prevent you from getting off the bed of nails you built. Loving yourself is in harmony with God's will for us.

Every painful event in my life had one common denominator, me. Bolts of lightning did not come down from the heavens and zap me. I had a part in the deal. With the help of my Higher Power, I can stop painful activity.

January 24

LIMITED VISION

Picture yourself in a prison cell, no windows, no light just four stone walls of darkness. Just one example of how limited our vision is to the bigger picture of what is happening in the universe. However, your personal Higher Power sees and knows all. In your morning meditation it is your time to communicate with the One who has limitless vision to help you with your narrow vision. Our world is what we can see and touch within an arm's length. It is the roof over our heads and a few meters around the neighborhood. When we were in our disease it limited our vision to the point of my example of a windowless prison cell. I was blind to the world.

Today my eyes are open and I accept my limits. In my morning meditation I connect with The Limitless One, my team mate for the game of life. I know only a little but I can increase my vision with the inspirations I get every day. The answers come because I ask for help. The only thing I am in charge of is my attitude. It is an attitude of gratitude and learning. I am a newcomer every day. Who is going to be my teacher today? Sometimes it is a new book, other times it is nature, a dog or a child. I am wide open to accept love and the messages of my environment.

When I go to an AA meeting, I receive the vision of about 20 fellow members who freely give me experiences and ideas of what to do and what not to do. This one hour expands my vision better than a set of binoculars. Priceless.

January 25

THE KINDNESS OF STRANGERS

The kindness of strangers is a wonderful and rewarding experience. My first trip to New York City I was prepared to meet rough, gruff treatment. Instead, when my friend and I hopped a taxi the super friendly driver saw we were in uniform. He drove us to a special hotel in the heart of city for military guys like us. Cost $1.

Then he said, "For you men in uniform, no charge, have a happy new year." This one gift of kindness led to a string of fortunate events including seeing a movie and the Rockettes on stage for free. The story of one stranger I never saw again.

In my role as a stranger, I wanted to do something of value on my amends trip through Vietnam in 2002. In the town of Dalat, I picked a high school student at random to support with a college scholarship. God led me to the right kid. Turns out he was the top student in high school so he had a great resume already. He could speak English, French, Chinese and Vietnamese. He secured entry at the University of Singapore and from there was able to get more scholarships all the way through a master's degree. A small act of random kindness caused positive ripples over the last 18 years. Today I look for more opportunities to be a stranger with loving kindness.

People like Mother Teresa and the Dalai Lama have spent an entire lifetime of loving kindness. We can learn so much from them. You too, can be the next stranger to change the world with loving kindness.

January 26

TO DISSECT IS TO KILL

I once read this description of a face, "eyes slanted upwards at odd angle, nose crooked, lips too wide and higher on one side." Who did this face belong to? An accident victim? No, it was describing Sofia Loren. The point is to dissect too much is to miss the beauty or even the meaning of the object. In biology class I was assigned to dissect a frog. Manual dexterity is not my strong point. The teacher looked at my work tray and inquired where my frog was. I pointed to the mess in front of me. My teacher advised me not to pursue a medical career. My patients would all die for sure. Once you dissect something it becomes unrecognizable.

When I was in Hawaii there was an AA study group that had a thirty-pound 1935 Webster's Dictionary to define each word in each sentence of the Big Book. I went to one session and they only covered one short sentence discussing the meaning in 1935 and how it would translate today. A gut-wrenching exercise. We call that "analysis paralysis" some people insist on. I enjoy the Big Book without dissection. God's harmony is to be enjoyed and dissecting anything kills the intent of the object like pulling the wings off a butterfly. It will never fly again and no one will see the beautiful colors float across their path.

I have faith when I flip on the light switch the darkness disappears and I do not need to have knowledge of electrical current. God does a thousand things for me every day and I don't have to ask why or how He does it.

January 27

UNDISCOVERED TREASURE

One of the Buddhist tales I think has a great message goes like this. "There was a young man who inherited substantial wealth from his father. One evening after falling drunk on the roadside, his friends took his wealth in gems. They sewed them inside his robe to prevent loss. The young man awoke in a fog and went around the village screaming he had been robbed. He spent the rest of his life in poverty begging for food in a homeless state. For years he possessed great wealth on his person but never knew it. He died a broken man." The lesson is all of us have hidden wealth we have not yet discovered.

More important than material wealth or special skills is discovering spiritual wealth. There is no upward limit to the spiritual awakening we have in our future. If I don't change, nothing is going to happen. I have learned through prayer and meditation I change for the better. New levels of spiritual awareness happen for me. It is a new horizon that should not be missed like the jewels sewed into your robe. The bright spot in our lives is showing others the great wealth they have within their grasp but they cannot see or even comprehend. We are so limited in our small world it takes some outside help to open the window to the rest of the universe.

We all have a treasure chest. Let the treasure hunt begin. I suggest prayer upon awakening for best results.

LOSSES

When we hit our bottom, most of us lost a whole list of things. I lost my house in a divorce, my car, my job and my future earnings. Just stuff. It was much worse to lose my health, self-esteem and self-respect. At the time I felt doomed to a life of misery. Now I realize I needed to lose everything to wake up. So many of the men I have worked with can't get past their losses. Most painful is the loss of a loved one but losing a million dollars hurts a lot too. I can truthfully tell my sponsees all my losses were replaced by following a spiritual path. Sobriety is the pot of gold at the end of the rainbow. Everything else will come later.

My bottom was deep, dark and painful. Just what the doctor ordered. All I had accumulated over fifty years went blowing in the wind. Perfect. I stood on a barren landscape with nothing. I was still alive despite my sickness. Enough life to see others before me had lost a lot but were happy. Sobriety turned their situations around and they promised the same could happen to me. It did. All those lost things on my list came back ten times over. All I had to do was surrender to the fact I needed to find a Higher Power and do the necessary steps for long term sobriety. There is nothing I had 27 years ago I miss or need. I gained a fortune.

I inventory my fortune every morning when I review my gratitude list. Nothing in the world is missing from my list. Now my task is to share it and give what I can to others.

I BELIEVE IT

A thought piece from Emmet Fox called, "The Dual Law of Thought," inspired me. His point being every thought has two factors, knowledge and feeling. Even a little bit of knowledge needs feeling to bring about action. If you believe your knowledge is true then you have the feeling to proceed. Many things are grooved into our thinking process as a belief. Short example, when I was a kid growing up, we were not allowed to go swimming for one hour after eating. We believed we would get cramps and drown if we violated the swimming rule. Turns out such a belief is false. I wasted hours of my youth. The point is what we believe may need a second opinion.

Once I entered into the world of recovery, I discovered so many of my old ideas were not only wrong but they were de-structive. Belief I could drink forever with no ill effects was almost fatal. Wrong. Everything was under control. Wrong. All my spiritual beliefs were fear based. Really wrong. Switching to love based spiritual beliefs was a complete reversal. It makes no difference if your knowledge is correct or not. What matters is what you believe to be true. I had to be re-born and start again from scratch.

God is Truth. What I think is truth is suspect. I need to connect with my Higher Power. Then I have a better shot at what is really true. Today I am willing to discard old beliefs and adopt a new path.

January 30

INSPIRATION AND PERSPIRATION

We all have heard faith without works is dead. Likewise, all the inspiration in the world does no good if we don't do the work. "God gave us the nuts but He doesn't crack them," a German proverb. I once saw a news show about a Betty Ford client who left the facility after 28 days and spent $40,000 then stopped at a bar on the way out and got drunk. He declared, "See it doesn't work." Amazing people think they can buy sobriety or have somebody else do the work necessary. There is a famous blog going around the internet called "Making My Bed". The point of the story is to start your day by doing something such as making your bed. A simple but positive first action.

Many folks make it to the rooms of AA and yet can't do what is required. In my own life I had a great work ethic reaping rewards for sweat and toil. I enjoyed working and seeing results for my effort. Doing the steps was a joy and continues to be delightful. I also was fortunate to be taught to do the whole nine yards, service, meetings, sponsor others, 12 step work, prayer, meditation, and inventory. I am grateful that my inspirations make my dreams come true and all I have to do is follow some simple steps with God's help.

There is no short cut to a new spiritual life our program offers. This is the easier softer way and I suggest just do the next right thing and pretty soon you will enjoy doing it.

Slip Prevention

Slip is too nice a word for losing sobriety. If I slip on the stairs it might kill me like it almost did seven years ago. If I take a drink it is just as dangerous as a tumble down the stairs. I guard against a slip every day without fail. I am not overconfident about my recovery. I know I must remain vigilant. Avoiding anger and resentments is tops on my priority list. I never declare myself "cured". Remaining teachable and viewing my program as a work in progress is my attitude. If I lose my balance of body, mind and spirit I am in danger. Taking time for fun and rest is important. With this virus it is easy to isolate but I try to keep in touch with the fellowship.

My sobriety is the most valuable thing in my life. My long gratitude list goes up in smoke with just one drink. I never had just one of anything. Becoming irritated over small stuff needs to be nipped in the bud. Losing one night's sleep upsets my entire system. I lose my compass and become negative. When I feel the slippery slope downward, I stop, drop and pray. My daily spiritual routine works well for me but events cause me to adjust. When this happens, I am extra careful not to have an emotional relapse. When I have fears I need to share them. Ignoring them doesn't work well for my sobriety.

Are you skipping meetings? Are you forgetting prayer and meditation? These are the questions I ask the guys I sponsor. I listen carefully to folks who have slipped. Ninety percent would answer my questions, "Yes".

February 1

WHAT ARE YOU GROWING UP THERE?

Another "law" from Emmet Fox caught my attention. The Law of Growth. His thesis is what you think upon grows. Your brain is like a little garden up there, growing mushrooms of either positive things or destructive thorn bushes. For example, when you have a resentment you form a mental list of the wrongs done to you, and a list of retaliation possibilities. You make another list of things to say to your enemy at the next opportunity. Your mind is growing stuff as you keep adding to all your lists. Growth on the positive side I see with my gratitude list. I can feel my gratitude garden growing up there and it leads to other happy thoughts expanding like crab grass.

The flip-side is those things you push out of your thinking atrophies into nothingness. I took calculus in school but after so many decades of non-use I could never solve a simple math problem today. I have to work hard to remember how bad it was at my bottom as the years push the nightmare out of my brain. The daily routine of reading and studying spiritual literature has grown over the years to the point it is foremost in my thought life. Negativity does not have a chance with me in the first hour of the morning. I water my garden every day.

What are you growing up there under your dome? The more you think of the good fortune already in your life, all the more good fortune will follow, says the Law of Growth.

THE TINY LITTLE VOICE

We all have a tiny little voice in our heads from time to time and whether we listen to it or not is key to our recovery. When I was drinking the voice was annoying and I would tell it to shut up. I turned up the volume to block the truth. Today a whole different story I not only listen carefully to the tiny voice but I trust what the voice says and follow the directions. My intuition is a combination of all my experience and years of being on a spiritual path. Every time I go against my intuition, I end up bruised. I don't care what conventional wisdom says or which way the crowd is headed. My intuition is the best path every time.

The tiny little voice tells me when to fold up and when to hold up. My intuition trumps fear and I press hard despite danger. When I have doubled down on authority like the IRS, law suits, etc. it has paid huge dividends. I know my Higher Power has my back when I am in a tense situation. Once we get sober, we get our brains back however scrambled. With restored intelligence and experience plus prayer we can face the world a lot better. Be confident God is on our side. The key is to get into action with what the little voice has to say. Good intentions die on the vine unless we take some risks and act with faith.

Intuition, inspiration, self-inventory, meditation and prayer in harmony make life exciting and positive. I listen to the tiny voice every day and try to tune out the other static. It takes practice and tenacity.

DON'T LOOK BACK

I can't stay sober on yesterday's meeting. Action today is needed to keep progressing in my recovery. I remember thinking my boss did not respect my accomplishments. I rattled off a list to which he just said, "OK Mike but what have you done lately?" Answer, nothing. I was sitting on my past looking back. We need to plow new fields and if you look at the farmer's plow it only works going forward. My spiritual teacher tells me Lot's wife was turned into a pillar of salt by looking back when instructed not to do so. An important message from the Bible. I get it.

Our AA Bible, the *Big Book*, tells us to move forward also. I tell the guys I work with to move through the steps as rapidly as possible and strive for some daily progress. For us, the past can drag down our progress. If we don't keep learning and growing, we are doomed. Knowing only a little makes me hungry for new opportunities to be of service, to help someone else, and open my mind to new thoughts. Once in a while someone will ask me about being a pilot. My pilot's license expired forty years ago. All the planes I ever flew are in the boneyard. I change the subject to a current reading of how to stay sober.

I keep my horizon clear for the unknown highways ahead. There is nothing I can do about all the ancient history of my past life. I can't afford the time to look back.

February 4

CARROT AND THE STICK

Remember the cartoon showing a rabbit with a carrot dangling from a stick too far to bite? Since the stick is attached to him the rabbit chases the carrot endlessly to no avail. The carrot and the stick are a way of life for me today. I set little positive goals in front of my face to entice my forward progress. There are service commitments to fill in just a few days' time and I want to make it. One more day of life above ground is a gift. Another day sober is a world's record for me. Each small goal or "carrot" gives me a sense of accomplishment. I feel useful and sometimes even victorious.

Yes, this a one day at a time program but some judicious planning for advancement and growth is a good idea. Leaning forward in the saddle will insure I don't fall into the past. There are people to see, books to read, books to write and a ton of carrots to put in my bushel basket. The carrot right in front of my face is my focus today. Once I grab the close one, I put a new carrot on my stick and I'm off to the races again. If I stop moving forward moss will grow under my feet. I will lose mobility. The goal is to be in heaven before the devil knows I am gone.

If I sit back in my rocking chair and watch History Channel soon, I will be history. Every day starts positive and I launch into the day with a fistful of tiny attainable goals.

February 5

APPLY THE BRAKES

One of the most enduring character traits you can adopt is one of self-restraint. The ability to keep your serenity and be still in the eye of an emotional storm is hard for some of us to master. This is a tough one for me as a Type A personality. I feel the need to be pro-active in every situation. I admire those who are cool with chaos all around them. People with Type B personality are just as effective as Type A. My point is you can leave things alone and enjoy a soft ride or you can stir up trouble of your own design and making. Backing off is not easy for me but I try.

Thinking things all the way through takes patience. Not my best attribute. If I can just hold myself back and let mistakes just happen and not reach out and try to gain control. I say to myself "Let go and let God," which quite often works better than counting to ten. God is the master planner and not every situation calls for my input. Another rule I say to my spinning brain is "Take every opportunity to keep my big mouth shut." Removing my hair trigger I carried around most of my life was key. A quick response to a negative barb thrown my way was my old way.

Restraint of tongue, pen and bad thoughts is my daily challenge. Doing nothing is always an option and at times the best option. If I close my eyes, I can hear my Higher Power saying, "Be still and know."

February 6

UNHATCHED EGGS

Most of us have laid some eggs of hope or projects never to come to life. They are just eggs of failure because nothing evolved. There are many eggs in my basket and my goal is to hatch some of them. The biggest success is my 4th Step egg. It laid around for a year, basically forgotten, until I got the life scared out of me. I finally sat on my egg until I did a complete and thorough moral inventory. Maybe the most important egg of my recovery. I had 2 eggs sitting in my living room for 3 years. Two sets of golf clubs I bought and never got out to the golf course to use them. As I look around there are books unread, music not played, cabinets not repaired. Yikes, a whole basket of unhatched eggs.

Many of us are prone to procrastination or just plain sloth, one of the deadly sins. The longer the egg just sits there, the harder the shell. For us in recovery we can inventory our egg collection and begin to hatch the more important ones. For some it is the 4th and 5th Step eggs and for some it is the 9th Step egg. Eventually they become rotten eggs from age and lack of care. All of us have projects "unhatched" but the 12 Steps need to come to life for our long-term sobriety. I have enjoyed hatching some eggs from before my drinking career. I have a few more in my basket.

Some dream projects may never be anything but a dinosaur egg. They might even turn to stone. In all of our inventories there is a golden egg needing attention. I am working on mine right now.

February 7

STOP ARGUING

In school I was on a debate team and it was enjoyable. Lots of rules and nobody raised their voice, pointed fingers or talked too long. As a drunk I lost the ability to be a gentleman in an argument and follow any rules of decorum. At the end I was arguing with myself, actually shouting and cursing. My first meeting taught me I did not have fight anybody or anything anymore. Arguing is kin to anger and resentment for me, since I can't remain cool-headed. Making my point shuts down any input from the other party. This mode is not communication but a one-sided rant. Arguing does not work for me, besides I'm not good at it anyway.

Some of my brothers in recovery relish argument and seek opportunities to push their agenda. If they get in my face, I just say, "Thank you for sharing." It has been years since I have been involved in a shouting match. A few people use the meeting to voice their argument with no interference from the opposition. I listen to their judgmental points, inventory taking and blame placement with quiet gratitude. I pray they feel better for venting their anger. Better in the rooms than out in the community. A foul mouth dissertation turns my stomach but it gives me the opportunity to set a different example in my sharing.

Arguing takes a lot of energy and often is destructive and negative. A peaceful discussion of differing ideas is possible but both parties need to be loving, open-minded and demonstrate serenity.

February 8

HOW TO BE ATTRACTIVE

One of the greatest aspects of our program is "attraction rather than promotion". We get peppered with promotion all the time and little of it lives up to the hype. Our program is "show me don't tell me." Everyone I ever helped was attracted to me before asking for help. I don't approach someone and suggest I should be their sponsor. First thing I learned early on from my AA grandma's is look the part of someone approachable. They taught me, "Mike you are not going to the beach. You shave, wear a shirt with a collar, show up early for meetings. You show that newcomer you care about this program." I have followed their advice for every one of the 10,000 meetings I have attended.

Presentable is not really attractive. What really makes you attractive to others is the person you are comes through by your words and actions in service. Add in a pleasant demeanor and a smile. A grouchy person is one most will stay away from even if they have 50 years sobriety. The fact you are the real deal is evident to those who know you. Your generosity with your time shows others you are approachable and available. When you share, it is your experience strength and hope. Not an angry tirade laced with foul language about your problems. If you are a happy person it can be contagious. A good sense of humor draws people closer.

If you have been on a spiritual path for some years the God within you will shine through to the outside. Other people will see it and feel it. You have my humble opinion on the secret to being attractive.

February 9

DOMINATION

In sports we hear statements like, "The Yankees dominated the bases and won the game 8 to 0." There will be another game tomorrow but what about being dominated personally? I hated being dominated but much of my working life I endured domination. I didn't like being controlled yet when I became a boss, I was a control freak. It was my turn to dominate. When you mix ego, power plays, and back stabbing to get ahead, look out. I lost a promising career by butting heads with someone who could dominate me. Then as much as I hated domination, King Alcohol took control of my life.

When we insist on dominating other people or situations it usually spells disaster. In AA if one person attempts to control the group, the group conscience neutralizes domination. On occasion we have to deal with bullies who push a certain agenda and the group retaliates. Sober alcoholics know domination first hand and they fight back. I never want to be dominated by anybody or anything ever again. My freedom from any type of bondage is precious. Domination has no place in AA or in my life. Also, I don't try to manipulate anyone. I hold my boundaries firm against unreasonable demands.

"Love does not dominate; it cultivates," quote from Goethe. In my relationships with others, I start with the principle we are all equal. I must love all my brothers and sisters.

February 10

GOD HAS A PLAN FOR YOU

Often, we hear God has a plan for every person. Our job is to seek God's will for us and align ourselves with the master plan. I knew for years I was in the wrong job in the wrong place. I felt trapped by circumstances. Twelve years into a military career I wanted out but felt I had too much time invested to quit. Sort of like throwing good money after bad. Then pour alcohol over the entire mess and automatically the picture is wrong. Even in the right profession in the right place alcoholism taints everything and spoils the soup.

One job out of the twenty different jobs I have been involved with lit my fire. One half of my day was teaching the principles of instruction to 16 students. Best feeling ever because I was giving of myself and I was good at it. The product was beneficial and it was fun. Getting sober was the beginning of aligning myself with God's plan. Although a novice, I became a writer. This sparked creativity and my writing is focused on helping others. Harmony has found me. I am doing the right things for the right reasons for the right people in the right place. I am confident I have found God's plan for me. I am supremely happy with life today.

Even though at an advanced age my heart is full of gratitude to reach this point in my life. At least I am blessed to have found it. So many of us never get there. My prayer for you is to find God's plan.

February 11

SLEEPING WITH THE ANGELS

Before I got sober sleep just wasn't a priority. Passing out does not count as sleep. Every night I would lie awake reviewing my resentments and listing the wrongs committed by my enemies. I would rehearse my plan of revenge. Afterwards came the fears of my behavior and possible troubles to come. No time for peaceful sleep. Today I am grateful for serenity and peace of mind. I sleep with the angels. The birds of worry have flown away. Daily problems are all luxury problems. I have no wish list, no bucket list, no want list. God has provided me all my needs and more. My brain can stop churning and spinning.

The first half of my life I ran my body into the ground. I never gave it proper care and rest. I viewed sleep as a waste of time when there was some excitement out there, I might be missing. Now I am so happy to be out of the excitement business. I cherish my sleep time. My days begin and end with prayer and it quiets the static of the daily buzz. If I am grateful and happy then tranquility follows. The absence of fear replaced by faith. Everything is going to be alright. God is the Conductor. The problems are out of my control. The actions of others, disasters and economy all are for God to handle.

Today sleep has a high priority. No stupid late-night movies or other time wasters. My sleep time is enjoyable and I am constantly healing from something. All kinds of magic are happening while I sleep with the angels.

THE HUMAN ANIMAL

Today's inspiration comes from the Dalai Lama. He suggests we learn our nature from the way our bodies are designed. If God intended for us to be aggressive animals, we would have large sharp teeth and a bigger mouth. He feels our human nature should be gentle. In addition, if we were meant to be jungle animals, we would have claws instead of hands and feet. I agree with the Dalai Lama. Our God given design gives us hints as to what our nature should be. Humans are the only animal with laughter and smiles. Our design and capabilities deliver a huge hint to the nature God intended for us.

Of course, we can act against our nature and be hurtful and play the part of a barnyard animal. To me the human body is God's work of art. Years of abuse and lack of proper care can smear the cosmetic beauty. The light of the heart and soul will shine through the rough exterior if we are in harmony with God's will. He has a plan for each of us. The body can take a tremendous beating, even the loss of some of the parts. It will still, carry us down the road of Happy Destiny. Wherever we have a weakness God gives us a strength in another area. I cannot hear well but I can see just fine.

God has forgiven me for my overall poor physical condition. In God's grace, He has left me enough equipment, albeit old and rusty, to act with the gentle nature He intended.

February 13

DON'T WORRY, DON'T HURRY

My spiritual teacher has offered four don'ts. Don't worry is a tough one for most of us. Worry is natural but when it consumes us, it becomes a problem. I worry about my kids, their safety and wellbeing. I know to let go and let them make their own mistakes without me trying to control them. My departed mother worried about the sad state of the entire world. She watched the news into the wee hours of the night wringing her hands and shaking her head in disgust. Most worry is really fear and it takes us out of the Sunlight of The Spirit. My teacher says, "You belong to God, and God is Love, so why fret?"

The second one is don't hurry. "Haste makes waste," I was taught from childhood. I was rushing all my adult life until recovery made me slow down. As soon as I was able to drive, I was a speeder, even though I had no reason to hurry. It was a habit of my entire life not only on the road but in all my activities. I have been in the slow lane for a few years now and I like it better. No more accidents, no more deadlines, I enjoy serenity. It is impossible to be tranquil if you are in a hurry. Emmet Fox says, "You are going to live forever, somewhere. In fact, you are in eternity now; so why rush?" Good way to look at it.

The other two don'ts on his list. Don't Condemn. Don't Resent. We all know resentments are the number one killer for us. "Don't worry, be happy," like the song suggests.

February 14

DEEPER RELATIONSHIPS

Most of us have hundreds of relationships but the majority of these are "surface" relationships. In other words, we know a lot of people by sight and greetings but nothing of their lives. Deeper relationships take some work on listening and empathy. I have been in a lot of fellowships and not many real friends have resulted until I joined AA. The difference is we share our emotions and inventory with each other. I remember family holiday dinners where all the men sat around the TV discussing the game. The women were in the kitchen talking about relationships and family problems. I enjoyed hanging around the kitchen much more until I got kicked out.

Everybody has a story but you will not ever hear the details until you go deeper than the game on TV. It takes some time to ask the right questions to learn more about someone. That's why resentments are stupid because you don't know enough about the other guy to judge him. If you knew more about what your adversary has been through maybe you would have more empathy. In fact, he might become a friend if you would open your mind and heart a bit more. Then there are the friends you already have but how deep is your relationship? What do you really know about their lives?

One of my daily prayers says it well, "To talk health, happiness, and prosperity to every person I meet. To make all my friends feel there is something in them."

February 15

ARROGANCE

On my list of topics to discuss is arrogance. I have never addressed this horrible defect of character. Hopefully I am out of the arrogance business. I don't like to think about it, talk about or write about it. Since humility is a key part of recovery then arrogance is the opposite in many ways. I have seen arrogance lead to relapse. In my inventory, I had an entire era of arrogance. Nothing more arrogant than an American fighter pilot. I tried to become the most arrogant of the arrogant. The war was over. I wasn't an active pilot anymore so my arrogant act quit working. It was fueled by alcohol and it was ugly.

In AA we have all seen the bleeding deacons with decades of sobriety preaching from a moral high ground. One member is heard saying to another member, "Hey dude, I have been sober a lot longer than you." Not good because we all only have 24 hours as the world's record. They forgot one of the two reasons we exist. "Stay sober and help other alcoholics achieve sobriety." Arrogance shows you think you are better than another. Such thinking goes against the entire grain of all my spiritual learning. Humility is being "right sized" and it is not in comparison to others.

"I spilled more booze on the bar than you ever drank." I find statements like this arrogant. I hope any trace of my arrogance has been removed because it certainly will not help anybody else. It turns people off.

February 16

LISTENING FOR THE QUIET

Hard to believe after an entire lifetime of noise I cherish quiet and seek it whenever I can. In the military it was all about noise. In combat if it gets quiet you can't sleep. In Thailand where I live it is noise 24/7 from all directions. Close to my condo is a bar that starts at midnight with a deep base thump, thump, until 5 a.m. My daily prayer and meditation begin about 5:30 a.m. when it is the quietest time of the day. No TV, no birds, dogs or human voices. Just me and my Higher Power so I can listen carefully. In my secret space there is no activity but prayer and peaceful quiet. I love my mornings.

Once I did a geographic to find a quieter place. After 3 months in Nong Khai, on the Mekong River I got the quiet I was seeking. But not enough AA meetings. Today I have a balance. I do get in the spiritual separation from the chaos of earthly surroundings and I fall into quiet sanctity of space. There is God waiting. My spiritual teacher tells me the most powerful prayer is, "Be still, and know that I am God." To me stillness and quiet are all part of deep meditation. When I am talking, I cannot receive the messages I need to hear. I suggest you hunt down a spot away from noise. Claim a secret cave for your next call to your Higher Power.

My favorite time is right before a meeting starts. All the drunks are loudly shooting off their yaps. Just before my headache begins the bell rings at 9 a.m. Silence. Thank You God.

February 17

LIFELONG FRIENDSHIP

I have been a newcomer for 27 years. Every day is a new benchmark of sobriety, a streak, a milestone. I hang with other newcomers and if they ask for help, I can form a true partnership. Fifty-fifty nobody is the boss or the best. Just two drunks with 24 hours starting at sunrise today. Most partnerships fail when one of the parties are no longer satisfied. When I stand next to someone, I am hoping it is not from any high ground. It is not a father-son relationship. We both have the same Father, God the Father. We are brothers in every sense of the word.

All of the guys I partnered with have become lifelong friends. I don't have all the answers but I have had great success with one alcoholic. Me. I share what worked for me. I print out the prayers I say. "Here my friend. Try these they have worked wonders for me." I show them what books I read and relate some gems I have picked up. I stress a gratitude list and provide a card to write one. I show my list to my partner, no secrets here. I never recommend something I haven't done myself first. Hopefully we both do step work together and enjoy the fruits of effort equally. The joy of seeing the lights come on to a once suffering soul is my reward.

A true partnership for us has to be about a spiritual path. No money, power or prestige involved. Two alcoholics involved in financial matters is always a disaster in my experience.

February 18

THE BREATH OF GOD

Every morning I pray for inspiration. The word inspiration comes from the Latin *inspirantio* which means "the breath of God." Every word I write comes from inspiration. God has answered my daily request for new inspiration. I try to carry the message of hope clearly and honestly. Inspiration does no good unless I put these thoughts into action. I never know where or when this inspiration will enter my conscious mind. I try to keep aware and awake for the blessings of my prayers to arrive. Sometimes an idea pops up from my spiritual readings. Today's inspiration came from a book on the craft of writing.

Most creative endeavors, such as writing, require inspiration to reach others in a positive way. The image of God's breath over my daily communication with my Higher Power is wonderful. I know my intuition and thought-life is in the right place. The closer to God I get, the stronger my intuitive voice. All the book knowledge in the world does me no good unless it sparks inspiration. Every morning I pray, read and meditate until I experience a spiritual awakening. God's breath in the form of heart talk, intuition and inspiration passes over me. This gives my mind and body the fuel for action.

I actively seek inspiration. God's nature never fails to provide. As my faith and trust in God grows, so does my inspiration.

February 19

Departure Plan

Are you ready for departure? Not next week. Right now, this minute. I see you grabbing your phone but where you are going there is no Wi-Fi connection. You have your ticket, it's been punched. Look at the destination. Ah ha, you are departing this life and entering a different non-material world. Look at your possessions, the car, the house, all will be useless. How about your family? They are not going with you. You might consider giving all your stuff to somebody you love. Do you have any resentments unresolved? Better clear those up because you won't get another chance. Debts to be paid? Nobody is going to clean up your inbox after you depart. You probably need to get busy.

We have talked about de-cluttering your life before. OK, it's show time. Do you have all your paperwork in one place for the loved one who will be saddled with the toughest part of your departure plan? I have a "croak" file with a will and government connections with my widow's benefits. If you really love who will be taking care of the mess you leave behind it might be prudent to be considerate of them. You can make it smooth as possible. To whom do you want to say, "I love you." Do it now. Last chance. Drop all your baggage this will be a weightless departure.

It is my belief my spirit will move on from my body. But my love will live on. Every night I say a departure prayer just like the arrival prayer I say every morning. I plan my departure to be without notice.

February 20

VALUABLE YOU

All of us are children of God and have some value by definition. How much value is largely up to us to determine. Being
rightsized is my way of estimating my value. I can't pretend
to be more than I am or lie about my accomplishments to seek
higher approval. I have discovered those who beat their own
drum are victims of low self-esteem. They feel they don't measure up. They create a false image with tall tales to back up the
mask they wear. Likewise, to hide one's talents under a bushel
basket is to deny the community at large the benefits of your
skill and expertise. If I remain right sized, my abilities are
available. My limitations keep me from blowing an empty
horn.

When I did my inventory, it became clear who I was and
who I was not. Ground zero. The idea is to increase my value
to be the best me I can possibly be. My prayers are for upward
goals and better character. My prayers are for repairing my past
by actions helpful to my fellows. I need not worry about what
value others place in me. If I have the respect of others that's
OK. If I don't it's OK also. I promise my Higher Power to
think only of the best, to work only for the best and expect only
the best. I can't cruise on past accomplishments. I need to act
today and guard against old behaviors.

I desire to speak the truth. I speak with love and the good
life we are blessed with. The value you put on yourself is the
one others will see.

A NEW LIFE

It takes a while to realize you have been given a new life. You have the same name but almost everything else has changed. Even your appearance is different now you are caring for your body. The miracle of recovery is just as dramatic as the parting of the Red Sea. A new set of principles. A new understanding of a Higher Power. A new action plan. New sober friends. New attitude. A new support group. An entirely new life. First, the old life must be torn down to the roots. You own your past, warts and all, learn the lessons then press forward. Second, you build a new life from scratch. One day at a time you build your new life with new materials.

This time you need not try to do it alone. Help is readily available from your Higher Power and the fellowship. This new life is a negative into a positive. Love based thinking instead of fears. Giving, as a way of life instead of taking. Thinking of others, instead of selfishness. A gratitude list to replace your wish and bucket list. Freedom from the bondage of resentments. You can now release all those bad guys in your brain. They were not paying rent. You can live in the now and drop the weight of the past. You can accept God's forgiveness as you forgive others. Once you discover who you really are, you can adjust your ego. Being right sized is much better than being less than or more than.

My new life compared to the old life is as different as black and white. Thank God I was blessed with a spiritual a-wakening into heaven on earth. I plan on doing my best with this second chance.

February 22

LOOK BEYOND THE HORIZON

When you are flying at 35,000 feet the radar will warn you of bad weather hundreds of miles over the horizon. Most of us live with just what we see in front of us, the immediate horizon. Our circle of movement is in a relatively small area so it is easy to forget what is over the horizon. My thinking goes over half the globe every day. I am in daily contact with my daughters exactly twelve time zones away so my 8 p.m. is their 8 a.m. They read my happenings in the morning and answer my mail before I sleep. The sun never sets on my family which I visualize as a circle of love across the oceans.

If you could look over the horizon and see all the AA meetings in all the different time zones going on right now it would boggle your mind. You can find a meeting in almost every country. Thanks to modern technology you can locate meetings all around the planet as you plan your travel. We are powerless but our fellowship is a positive force worldwide. In my small town my meeting has increased 400% in ten years. In Thailand the number of Thai AA members you could count on one hand ten years ago. Today there are several hundred Thai AA members. Also, over twenty Thai language meetings. It has been a great joy to watch the growth and be part of it.

I am blessed to sponsor several men half way across the world. We are as close as two brothers can be. AA will continue to grow as new technology shrinks our world to a heartbeat away.

POCKETS OF ENTHUSIASM

Years ago, I heard a speaker talk about "pockets of enthusiasm". His theme came to mind during my morning meditation. I realized I was in the middle of one of those pockets he was talking about. I spent all weekend with 200 members of AA from 26 different countries. There was something special and electric about the atmosphere. Of course, all of us had a lot in common as recovering alcoholics but it was something higher up. The love and the laughter made the air sweeter. So many friends who only see each other once a year. It was like a family reunion on steroids.

At this event I was in service. As I observed all the other folks in service, it hit me. The spark running the love machine was from my home group. I could readily identify the core of enthusiasm. My home group has been on my gratitude list for 15 years but this weekend gave me a spiritual awakening. I live daily in the pocket of a special group arguably the best in Thailand. It has been my good fortune to be a trusted servant for so many years. Just one of the bozos in the back row with a bunch of clowns of the same mind. The special "something" has attracted others to a standing room only crowd.

My heart was so full of gratitude as I realized I was experiencing a new plateau. It is something spiritual with a multiplier effect of increased love and appreciation for each other.

February 24

ABSOLUTE HONESTY

Our founders stressed the importance of honesty. When we were practicing our disease, honesty was not a priority. We lied to cover up our behavior. The biggest lies were the ones we told ourselves. I can handle my drinking. A lie. I'm in control of my life. A lie. I'm not hurting anybody. A lie. The truth escaped us. We lost a grip on reality. We created a fantasy existence. I know I lost the ability to separate fact from fiction. My web of lies became too complicated to sort out. My inventory exposed my dishonesty to the light of day. My lying was a habit hard to break.

Achieving absolute honesty was a tough challenge when I entered recovery. I didn't even know who I was. It was like entering kindergarten to recognize right from wrong. To be honest with others, trust is required. I had no trust. When I started attending meetings, I could feel the honesty in the sharing. I was able to follow their example. Slowly, I trusted myself. I stopped lying to myself and others. Doing my fifth step with my sponsor was two days of honesty. It felt good. I felt right inside my gut for the first time in decades. The truth has set me free.

My lies came in the form of rationalization, exaggeration and denial. Rigorous self-honesty is essential to my recovery and spiritual growth today.

February 25

... AND MEAN IT

My spiritual teacher has given me a new idea to add to my mantra as I do my daily routine. For example, from this prayer called "Life Is a Celebration" a few lines go like this: Encourage another...and mean it. Keep a promise...and mean it. Show my gratitude...and mean it. Yes, I enjoy saying my prayers but do I really plan on turning them into concrete action? It is so routine my concentration is not always attuned. Lately I have slowed my pace down and after every line I say to myself...and mean it. I want my prayers to change me and not be hot air.

My spiritual guru suggests another kind of diet. A mental diet. His point is we become what we think and concentrate on. What we read and listen to is the mental food we consume every day. Those daily prayers are a regular part of my mental diet. I wrote about really meaning those words going in to my brain. My daily readings, again require a slow pace to think about the message contained in my mental intake. Subtracting news programs and stupid movies is a great mental diet. Staying away from negative people who talk hate and discontent spices up my mental diet. I enjoy fun people instead.

I am what I eat and what I think. Watching what is entering my body and mind needs careful filtering. This new diet I am working on sounds great. I will do it...and I mean it.

February 26

THE PATH OF LOVE

Love is the answer. This I truly believe. The path of love is open to everyone. No special skills or high intellect required. God is Love so if we seek God on a regular basis we are on the right path. Love is a positive powerful force. Since we know we are powerless then why not tap into a never-ending power source—love. In my previous life I thought the path of action was my best option. I decided to fight for my place to the top. For a time, it worked but it was such hard work to fight constantly. Love is gentle.

I will never forget the first time I heard in a meeting, "You don't have to fight anyone or anything anymore." I realized I had the wrong approach to life all along. Love is much easier than fighting I promise you. We know God loves us and wants the best for us. All we need to do is continually seek God and His will for us. If God is within each of us then love resides inside each of us also. It is a natural part of our being. We need to find ways to express this God given love in our daily life and actions. Going through a divorce sounds like the opposite of love but it does not have to be. Right after I got sober, I experienced a loving divorce. All parties were satisfied and went our separate ways with love.

I try to apply the love solution to all my problems these days and it works. I know the path of love is right for me.

February 27

GET OUT OF JAIL FREE

With a glass of booze in my hand, I had a moment of clarity. All of a sudden, I realized I was imprisoned. I had food, drink and bathroom privileges. But I could not go anywhere. I lived too far to walk anywhere and it was too dangerous to drive and risk a DUI. The door was open to freedom but I had a ball and chain. I had no way out, no options, no future and no clue. If I only knew how wonderful life could have been if I would just have given up and surrendered. I was isolated, lonely and defeated. If I only knew freedom was a phone call away. I am grateful for a set of events that drove me to AA and a rebirth.

Now we have freedom on our gratitude list how about other "jails" we have in our inventory? Have we locked ourselves out of important progress? We are in charge of our own limitations and often we underestimate ourselves. We may not be totally free even though the door has been opened. Now because of our new way of life we have a "get out of jail free" card. It may be a great time to cash it in. If there is a door in front of you, I suggest you try it. You might find it open. If the door is locked, God has opened a window somewhere. You just have to find it.

I leave you with this prayer, "Dear God, inspire me to send my roots deep into the soil of life's enduring values. May I grow toward the stars of my great destiny."

February 28

CAUSE AND EFFECT

We often hear in meetings, "I don't have a drinking problem, I have a thinking problem." Actually, a very wise statement. Emmet Fox says, "Mind is cause, and experience is effect. If you do not like the experience or effect that you are getting, the obvious remedy is to alter the cause and then the effect will naturally alter too." All of us reached the point the effect of drinking was no longer acceptable. We needed to change our minds, the cause. After decades of ingesting mind-altering substances our minds were distorted. An undesirable effect was inevitable. After all those years of wrong thinking I need a daily dose of spiritual thinking and direction.

Our minds set us apart from other animals as a superior kind of animal. Our habits of thought determine our character and our actions. Only my own thoughts can put me in bondage. On the flip side, my happiness comes from the cause, my own mind. I can control my thought life to make contact with my Higher Power who has all power. All I have to do is ask and pray as my means of communication. I love the effect. Any time I am not satisfied with the effect of my daily living I can go back to the cause and adjust my thinking patterns.

One thing I can control is my attitude which formulates my thought life. If I have an attitude of gratitude then the effect is always happy joyous and free. I pray every day for the courage to change my thinking for the better.

February 29

START WITH A PLUS SIGN

The power of positive thinking can never be underestimated. When faced with a difficult problem there is always positive and negative aspects. If you can connect one positive portion of the problem to another you may have a chain of stepping stones to a better result. For example, divorce, which is negative by its very nature. Feelings are wounded all around and emotions run high. Most likely both parties feel like they are not getting their fair share of the pie during the breakup. Forget the pie for a while and find the plus sign. Children are a good positive spot of common ground. Communication can start with the welfare of the children. This focuses on something outside of the couple. Now build a dialogue from one plus sign.

OK now we have start, then it takes some loving attitudes to continue. I have found humor to be a big ice breaker. A good laugh breaks down hostility and all parties have a smile on their faces. It releases tension. The next step is to mentally play the part of the other person and try to argue their point instead of yours. Think about their fears and pull a plus sign out of their argument. You can begin your next sentence with, "I agree with you about this point." Of course, saying nothing might be your best positive action. Just smile and give your opponent a hug. Love is the answer.

In your morning meditation, ask your Higher Power for the right path on difficulties. If you start your day with a few plus signs, there is a good chance you can stay positive.

March 1

PERSISTENCE

Our path is one of persistence and faith. When problems are nipping at our heels it is hard not to get distracted and lose our temper. Prayer is not a stop and start deal. It is continuing as a regular practice. Our prayers will be answered but not how and when we envision. Our field of view is so limited but God's view is all knowing, all understanding. It took many years to get us to a bottom thus many more years will be required to climb out of the hole we have dug for ourselves. I know I persistently drank. Now I must persistently practice my recovery routine and remember this is "slowbriety".

Only Divine Providence made us put the glass down. Only Divine Providence can lead us to repair the damage. We can become a useful member of society again. The best way to connect with our Higher Power is prayer and most of us have concrete examples of prayer working. All we have to do is be persistent in our prayers. Don't give up before the miracle. These prayers will work if they come from the heart. Meaningful sincere prayers are going to help you through your difficulties. They will keep you in a positive frame of mind. We should have no doubts. If we turn our life over to our Higher Power, He will see us through. Keep the faith.

On our path we will have peaks and valleys, setbacks but steady progress. Be persistent. If you get impatient or discouraged just think back to the days you were drinking up to your ass in alligators.

March 2

WHY OUR ORGANIZATION WORKS

The outside world is amazed at the success of AA. No president, no rank structure, no fees or dues, no super stars. Sounds impossible but we know how it has grown. First of all, our fellowship is love based whereas so many other organizations are fear based. My life in the military was fear based. The reason we have a military at all is the fear of losing our territory or our ideals. I know I spent a lot of time fearing death with people trying to shoot me down. AA has no police, no punishment, no rules only "suggestions". You cannot be expelled or thrown out of our fellowship. It is totally about giving and not focused on taking.

Buddha makes types of organizations quite simple.

1. One based on power, wealth or authority of great leaders

2. One based on convenience to the members and will continue as long as the members remain satisfied and do not quarrel.

3. One based on good teaching as its center and harmony is its very life.

OK, Buddha we will take Door #3 as our organization type.

In AA we have one product, sobriety. You can't buy it by the can or bottle. No warehouse is required. We have a spiritual base and stress unity, love and harmony. It works.

GOD AS WE DON'T UNDERSTAND HIM

We always talk about the "God of our understanding" in our program but in reality, none of us understands God. My "understanding" is a fluid, growing thing ever changing over time. I continue my pursuit of God's will and guidance. My spiritual teacher has listed some main aspects of God. First of all, God is Life. Just look at all the many parts of the body, a Grand Design by a Supreme Being. God is Truth. God is not truthful but Truth itself, and wherever there is Truth, there is God. God is Love. I truly believe God loves us and His love is there when we need it. All we have to do is ask through prayer. I know when I feel God's love, I fear nothing at all.

My teacher goes on to say God is Intelligence. Easy for me to accept. I know only a little but God is all knowing. It makes me go to Him for enlightenment. I need to do His will. God is Soul. When you are called upon to perform some task too great for you, realize you are one with God. The task will become "our business" instead of "my business." God is Spirit. Spirit cannot be destroyed or damaged. Your true spirit was never born and will never die. It goes on after the body decays. Finally, God is Principle. In other words, we cannot pray for the laws of gravity to be set aside. We cannot leap over tall buildings.

All these aspects are difficult to understand. The many attributes of God such as truth, wisdom, beauty, love, and joy are compounds of several aspects. I remain in awe of my Higher Power as I try to understand Him.

March 4

OPEN SESAME

How open is your mind? It is a basic human trait to resist change. Most of us have made the biggest change of all. The change of a knee walking drunk into a sober useful member of society. I am grateful for the transformation of a lifetime. Once again, I have become a creature of habit to maintain my sobriety. I do all the things I was taught to achieve long term sobriety and it works well for me. I have a good routine but maybe something is better to replace good. Wouldn't it be nice to just shout "open sesame" and let new ideas flow in for a fresh change of pace? Recovery memory sort of like muscle memory.

Lately I have been reading articles to improve my writing. I have been making the same mistakes and misspellings for decades. The door I am trying to open has rusty hinges. At least I know I need improvement and am open to changing my bad habits. The proof of my efforts will be evident in my writings. For my recovery and my writing, I look for new information and remain teachable. Humility mixed in with an open mind is key to dropping a know-it-all attitude. Being an old newcomer is a way of life for me today. I make an effort to think "out of the box" and ask for help when necessary.

The point is to be willing to accept new thoughts, new information and avoid a rut. Even when things are going well, I know if I stay on the same track I will get run over. I need to keep moving.

CONFESSIONS OF A RUNNER

True confession, yes, I have been a runner all my life. Not being able to handle confrontations well, my solution was to run. As a kid my only athletic ability was running. Going the mile back and forth to school I often had to run to avoid gang areas. Dressed in Catholic school uniform I was easy pickings for lunch money. I ran away from home three times before it worked. The truth be told I joined the military because I was running away from parents and my messes. I was able to use the military way of life to run away from bad jobs and relationships. Eventually they gave me an airplane. Now I could not only run away, I could fly away.

One unforgettable escape I was in my aircraft running away from a relationship where I had been hurtful. I was so happy to be free. When I caught my image in my tail view mirror, I saw a deceitful liar looking back. Like a ton of bricks, I realized I was not escaping at all. I could not get away from me. I was transporting the problem very fast and far but running was not a solution. All I did was relocate the problem. It was a moment of clarity seared into my conscience. My first AA meeting when I saw all the happy laughing group, I was ready to run away. My soon-to-be sponsor grabbed my arm tight and said, "You are in the right place."

He was right of course, I stayed for the miracle. Some folks doing my inventory thought I ran away to Thailand. This time I ran to a giving, loving culture to replace the taking culture I left behind. I am too tired to run anymore.

March 6

LIFESTYLE

One of my readings suggested comparing my lifestyle as it is today against my drinking lifestyle. I did and it gave me an overwhelming feeling of gratitude. The difference is like night and day. Black and white. Happy and unhappy. The time before I got sober life was a struggle, a fight. My bar had every known type of alcohol. Anything less would be unacceptable. Looking back, I was all style and no life. In the end, my private club had only one member, me. I was in charge until the truth bubbled to the surface. My inventory showed my lifestyle before recovery was all about material wealth, power and prestige. It was completely devoid of anything spiritual.

Once I got on the road to a sober lifestyle the change was total. My old ways did not work and the new ways did. It became more about life and not style. Living each day to the fullest and asking God for help every morning brought humility and gratitude. My purpose in life went from self-serving to serving others. I stopped collecting "stuff" and stripped down my possessions to the basics. I stopped trying to impress others and impressed myself with my spiritual progress. My old "power" was smoke and mirrors. My Higher Power has a new resource opening a whole new life for me. Today I have a real life and a simple style.

The secret to a wonderful life style is removing me from the material world. Now it is one day at a time into the spiritual world. Simple.

March 7

SPECTATOR OR PARTICIPANT?

At most sporting events there are a few players on the field and a lot of spectators in the bleachers. The players have all the action and the spectators sit on their butts and pass judgment on the players. Meanwhile the players take all the risks and injuries. In my experience so goes life in organizations. There are pluses and minuses in both roles. Ask yourself if you are a spectator or a participant in service to AA? It appears to me, AA is just like many other organizations. A handful of trusted servants open up, set up and clean up. The majority come expecting everything to be ready for them, they drink coffee and complain.

I was given tasks to perform in service to my family as soon as I could walk. I worked my way through high school. Then I spent 30 years in service to my country, a good fit for me. In the military I was in the 10% of action players at the tip of the spear. I have been judged, criticized and threatened in my years of being a participant. It never stopped me from pressing on. I am not saying being a participant is better than being a spectator. I admire the folks who don't get into action. I don't understand how they can sit on the sidelines. What a gift. For me, the benefits of being in action and service in AA are too great to be missed.

Getting involved makes you part of the process versus an observer. Commitment is better served by action. Maybe a minority opinion. It is up to you.

THE LAW OF SUBSTITUTION

We all know about substitution, after all we substituted recovery for our drinking. We found new uses of our time to replace the void when we put down the drink. So why not apply substitution in our thought life? Our brain works best in quiet relaxed ways not by strain. When we press hard on our brain, we get a headache and zero solutions. That is why a morning of quiet meditation is so important to our recovery. I hear people say, "I am struggling with this problem," when they should be saying, "I have given my problem over to my Higher Power." The solution has to come from outside your limited thought process.

One true story example of "substitution" is the saga of Bat 21 in the Vietnam War. Bat 21 got shot down and was in enemy territory. He was able to facilitate his rescue by comparing his location to his home golf course. The rescuers were able to save his life by this "out of the box" solution. In my own case, I "substituted" a gun butt for a wrench to open a gas barrel to refuel my downed aircraft. I prayed to my Higher Power and He provided the assist because I had no clue. If you substitute your thoughts, negative to positive, a solution you would never think of will present itself. I can control my thoughts and do a substitution if necessary.

"We know that thought control is the key of destiny, and in order to learn thought control we have to know and understand these laws," quote from Emmet Fox. The law of substitution is just one.

SLEEP ON IT

We pause—and wait. Such a good idea when hit with a volatile situation. It is not easy for us alcoholics to be quiet and consider all the aspects of a bad encounter. It would be better to sleep on events. There isn't much out there requiring a firebrand response. My mouth can get me in so much trouble and once it leaves my lips it is on the street forever. Why do I think I am in charge of every situation and not ask my Higher Power for help? I try to remember the GAP, God Authorized Pause. It's OK to hesitate and think things through. I try not to get ahead of God and be in a big hurry to be wrong.

It is simple really. God has all Knowledge and all Power and I do not. I just need to think of God in times of stress and when faced with hostile people and situations. Why not sleep on it, cool off and rest my spinning brain? In my morning meditation, I am turning it over to my best friend, my partner, my Higher Power. I need to let my heart have the podium and come up with a calm, loving plan of action. Maybe no action is best. When I am angry my vision is blurred and I don't see what is important. I only see red and lose the black and white in front of me. "All things pass...Patience attains all that it strives for," quote from St. Teresa of Avila.

Talking to a sponsor or a good AA friend will always cool your fire and give you a different view point. At least it will slow you down. Give your difficulties to God and get out of the way.

HOW TO EXTEND YOUR PAIN

Part of life is pain and suffering as we all know. Buddhist teaching has many lessons concerning the problems dealing with the inevitable pain of living. My favorite author about pain and illness is Emmet Fox. He has a whole chapter titled "How to Destroy Your Health". His point is we extend our pain by focusing on the illness and talking about your problems to others. We tend to rehearse our sad tale for others to empathize and share the misery. His remedy is to think of God and all aspects of God. Your body is the Temple of the Holy Spirit. To not recognize this fact is to go against God and then we are headed for still more trouble.

I read several spiritual discussions about pain and suffering. I had many opportunities to put the teachings to the acid test. It works. I had several operations and procedures in recent history. There it is, history to be in a chart on file in my doctor's office. I do not talk about these events anymore. I have a bad knee, it aches all the time if I focus on my knee. It is just aching away without bothering me as I go about life. At my age everything is rusty and all the parts are used to the breaking point. Sooner or later a part or two is going to break. I am OK with pain as an opportunity.

In my extensive survival training I was taught the body will shut down automatically at too high a pain level. So why worry? Relax, get sleep so the body can heal itself without you having to think about it.

THE KINGDOM OF GOD IS WITHIN YOU

We all know stories of great pilgrimages seeking God and Truth. God is within us and a worldwide search is not necessary. Our consciousness is where a Spiritual Awakening can and will take place. It is so important to understand all those Laws of Practice, Growth, Forgiveness, Relaxation and Subconscious Activity. These are like the law of gravity, what goes up must come down. It goes with all these laws of the conscience mind and control of our thinking. The harmony of all these working in concert is where we connect with our Higher Power. We can find our destiny and become the beautiful person God intended for us to be.

I know I must change the person I was when I was drinking and become a useful human being. I accept my powerlessness and know the only thing I can control is my attitude and my thoughts. I can remove my negative thinking for positive ones and enlist the help of my Higher Power. My morning prayer fills my heart and my head with nothing but positive input. I always have a good start. God is with me every day and I can call on His help by simply asking through prayer. The Kingdom is available and all I need to do is seek God's will for me. God will do for me what I cannot do for myself.

We can find happiness by right thinking and seeking the God of our understanding inside our own hearts. If we feed our mind, body and spirit with the right stuff we can stay on the Road of Happy Destiny.

March 12

CRITICISM

Nobody likes a critic. I remember two movie critics on TV years ago. They were arrogant and nasty. Their job was to judge movies but people who criticize others are just as distasteful. Most alcoholics share my disdain for critics. I know of no one who got sober by being criticized. The program of recovery allowed me to do my own inventory. My sponsor did not laugh at me or poke fun at my failings when I did my fifth step. I could see my faults clearly. My character defects became obvious. I saw no need for someone else to pour salt in my wounds.

Likewise, I am not a critic. There are loving ways to suggest a different path to someone in danger. When working with others I want to help, not hurt. I have never been a fan of "tough love". My suggestions to others are framed in terms of my own experience. The man I am trying to help can connect the dots. The solution to his problems has to be his idea not mine. Being critical involves judgment. It infers I know better. Since we are all equal, I don't place myself higher and judge. I talk to others the way I like them to speak to me. On rare occasions, constructive criticism may be necessary.

If I get criticized, I let it roll off my back. The judgment of others is out of my control. Rather than fight back, I let them keep their opinion without challenge. I don't have to engage.

March 13

CHOICES

Another key item on my gratitude list is freedom of choice. The cycle of life shows a beginning with no choices. A big window of time where we do have choices. In the end all the choices are lost as we pass. Your first awareness is somebody caring and making choices for you. They fed you strained peas. You didn't choose your parents, the color of your skin or your location. Slowly you grow into choice making. We choose our life's work, our mates, and to change our location. Unfortunately, we choose to drink and drug to the point of near destruction. A choice we all have in common. We sought help and chose recovery over death.

Now on the road to recovery we have the ability to make wiser choices. At my bottom, I had no more choices, I had to drink. I was immobile. What a wonderful gift to wake up to dozens of choices each day. Most of my choices are easy to make. Feed my brain with spiritual readings and prayer. Feed my body with good nutritious food, and exercise. Be in service. Then with the tough choices, I can ask for help from my Higher Power and my trusted friends. As the body slows with age, choices are limited for mobility and maybe back to strained peas.

We seek to do the next right thing. We seek to make choices in harmony with our spiritual path. Along with this wonderful freedom comes the responsibility to be loving, giving and positive.

March 14

THE LAW OF GROWTH

This is another in the series about thought control. This law is very easy to understand. Whatever thoughts you have, good or bad, grow as you think on a particular subject. For example, a thought enters your mind, Joe. Then you start thinking about Joe who has insulted you. You don't like Joe. He is a mean and vicious person in your opinion. He has done the following dozen things to hurt you. Your negative thought grows and may even bring you to action. In my days of harboring resentments, I would lay awake at night listing all my points over and over. If I only knew the Law of Growth back then I might have been able to sleep.

Whatever you think upon grows says the Law of Growth. The more you think of the good fortune you have, the better fortune will come to you. The gratitude list I keep talking about is key to your thought control to channel your growth in a positive direction. Just one thought leads to a chain of thoughts as our mind concentrates on a particular subject. We get to choose our thoughts. We can nip anger in the bud when a weed starts to grow. The more injustices you think about the more will follow you. The more you concentrate on your blessings more good things will be yours. The outside world has a lot of negativity. The task is not an easy one.

Your morning visit with your Higher Power grows every day in a loving forward-looking manner. The stronger the morning routine gets the better your growth patterns.

The Law of Forgiveness

Our 11th Step Prayer addresses forgiveness for our thoughts, "It is by forgiving that one is forgiven." The Lord's Prayer has forgiveness in the heart of the message. "And forgive us our trespasses, as we forgive those who trespass against us." Most spiritual teachers will stress the importance of forgiveness as a necessary step to lasting inner peace. The USA turned their back on Vietnam and Laos. I still feel the pain. Have I accepted what happened? Yes, but the fact I am even writing about it shows I have not really forgiven my country. In fact, I don't live there. I have a lot of forgiveness work yet to do.

The Law says, "You have to forgive others if you want to demonstrate over your difficulties and make any real spiritual progress." I hear people say, "OK I can forgive but I will not forget." Not good. You can forgive in words but if you refuse to forget about it then you really have not forgiven. I have forgiven family members for what they have done. I can still recall the incidents and rewind them for you. Not really forgiveness. Once it is out of my thought process forever then I can totally render forgiveness. Resentment, condemnation, anger, desire to see someone punished are things rotting your soul. Such things fasten troubles to you with rivets.

Emmet Fox writes, "You must forgive injuries, not just in words, or as a matter of form, but in your heart—and that is the long and short of it. You do this, not for the other person's sake but for your own sake."

March 16

GENEROSITY

Generosity was not part of my life until well into my recovery. Selfishness was the order of the day until I woke up to a spiritual life. To combat my selfish nature, I learned to focus on giving instead of taking. My daily prayers are all about giving to others. This gold mine I tapped into must be shared. The basic culture of Thai people is to give anything they have. Even homeless Thai folks will offer food from their plate if you happen to pass by. One of the reasons I live here. I have reprogrammed myself to look for ways to be generous. Anonymity is part of the deal. I don't want an award for whatever I give. Ego should be removed from a generous act.

A friend recently told me about all the old clothes and furniture he donated to a church. He said it felt good to be generous plus he got a tax deduction. I agree being generous feels good. The tax benefit makes the whole thing a wash. Generosity means giving of yourself more than money or stuff. Your time has value. Being present to lift some boxes for a friend moving has value. Just sitting by a hospital bed to comfort a person on a respirator is generosity. An act of love has no strings attached. I love you but you need not love me back. Generosity from the heart is love.

My friend, the Dalai Lama says there are three types of generosity: material aid, spiritual teaching and protection from fear. Whatever I give in love I receive much more in spirit.

Returning Your Spirit on Departure

My spiritual teachers all stress the fact the spirit is not born and does not die. We as spiritual beings have a spirit within us while we are alive. Once our body dies our spirit goes on into eternity. With this in mind, I was inspired by one of my favorite Native American prayers titled, "Oh Great Spirit. Make me always ready to come to You with clean hands and straight eyes. So, when life fades, as the fading sunset, my spirit may come to You without shame." Body, mind and spirit all need our loving care as God's gift to us while we are alive. Whoever had my spirit before me did a great job. I need to do the very best for my spirit before I present it back to God.

I am so grateful I didn't pass away drunk in the gutter somewhere. The care for my spirit was zero until I put down the drink for the last time and surrendered. Blessed indeed this is a spiritual program. My spirit was in such poor repair it needed immediate attention for my recovery. My hands were dirty and I could not look anybody in the eye, including myself. Today I work diligently on my spiritual condition knowing full well perfection is not possible. My life today has a spiritual center. My mind and my body are fading quickly. At least I can keep my spirit strong.

When I pass, my spirit will go on. I see my task is to do the best job possible to return my spirit with more knowledge and improvements. I am blessed to get 80 years to do the job right.

March 18

LAW OF PRACTICE

This is the last of the series on Laws for our thought life. Practice is probably the easiest to understand. We become what we practice. If you examine all the super stars in sports it is no secret practice and more practice equals success. Andre Agassi discussed how he hated tennis and was forced to hit 1500 balls every day. He became a super star but at some personal cost. You can be good at cooking, welding, artwork, playing a piano just by years of practice. The Law states practice is the price for proficiency. There is no achievement without practice and provided it is done intelligently, the greater the proficiency.

In our quest for thought control it is just a matter of intelligent practice. If we find what works and do it repeatedly, we will achieve our goals. In AA we have that written in Step 12, "to practice these principles in all our affairs." OK what are these principles? Self-honesty, Hope, Faith, Courage, Integrity, Willingness, Humility, Self-discipline, Love, Perseverance, Spiritual Awareness, and Service. If we do these every day to the best of our ability then we achieve long term sobriety. We are not ever going to be perfect but we should try to be the best person possible. In our meditation, we enlist the help of One Who is All Perfect.

When I review my gratitude list, I can see the fruits of my daily practice. I achieved the desired goal of not only staying sober but I can now help others. I can be happy, joyous and free.

March 19

PROGRESSIVE

Once life becomes good again it would be wonderful to stop right there. But we can't make the world stop when and where we like. Everything is progressive. Life is progressive. Our disease is progressive. We have been taught we have a daily reprieve contingent on our spiritual condition. It is hard to imagine as each day passes, our disease became worse. True, we didn't drink but our disease progresses as if we did drink. I witnessed several members take a drink after 20 or 30 years of sobriety. Once they took the first drink their bottom came with the speed of light. They never could recapture the fun. This disease tells me I am OK but it is not the truth. If I could visualize my disease like an expanding rash, I would see the truth.

The good news is our spiritual condition is progressive. If we take our daily medicine we can stay out of danger. Prayer builds on more prayer. Your connection with your Higher Power improves when you stay vigilant and persistent. You have the power to improve your mind, body and spirit. You can extend your life through good care and intelligent choices. I desire more spiritual progress. I need to stay alive to reach my goals of more amends, more love and good works. Death ends progression. To drink is to die just like the *Big Book* promises. Progression is a good thing as long as I maintain my spiritual recovery.

I know only a little. At my present rate of progress, I will be considered "wise" in 300 years. As long as I tap the wisdom of my Higher Power I need not worry about progression.

March 20

COMPASSION

Most religions have one basic rule. Love one another. Why is this simple principle so hard to follow? Fear instead of love seems to rule so much of our lives. My buddy, the Dalai Lama, has much to say about compassion in his writings. Real compassion is feeling the suffering of others as if it were my own. If my brother is ill, then I too am ill, to some extent. If we speak of compassion but have no action to go with the words, it is just hot air. If our action is not from the heart it is not true compassion. Real compassion comes up from our hearts into words and action.

The Dalai Lama goes even deeper to say even if your compassion is rejected it does not change true compassion. We can relate when we offer help to the still suffering alcoholic and he refuses the helping hand. We still keep our compassion strong. In the same vein, compassion brings us happiness as part of an attitude of loving kindness. The Dalai Lama says, "The more compassionate, kind and gentle a person, the more he or she should be respected." With true compassion comes a sense of responsibility and the desire to help your brothers and sisters. Intimacy and compassion weave together in a tapestry of love.

My study of compassion leads me to believe it is a personal matter of the heart. I work to push away from selfishness. I can feel my level of compassion and tolerance grow.

March 21

WHICH DO YOU FEED?

All of us have a good side and a bad side. Positive and negative. I think about the Native American Indian fable about the two wolves. The old chieftain is teaching his grandson some lessons of life. The old sage tells his grandson that we all have two wolves in our hearts. One white wolf who is kind, sharing and strong. The other black wolf is mean, selfish and evil. "Grandson only one wolf can survive in your heart." The young boy asks, "Grandfather which wolf will survive?" The chief replies, "Only the one you feed." I stress meditation to feed your good side with nothing but positive, spiritual inputs.

If we want to nurture a God centered conscience then it stands to reason our inputs will help the process along. The wrong inputs will stop progress and even reverse our recovery. If I frequent bars and participate in all the bar activities, even without the alcohol, I am practicing old behaviors. I'm not "feeding" anything useful. We all have a Mr. Hyde inside of us. Now I try to be one person and starve Mr. Hyde from my personality. Treating all persons with loving kindness and respect is actually much easier to manage. I feed my brain daily with good healthy inputs. I keep my attitude in tip top shape.

As an alcoholic I need to curb anger, fear and resentments in a different way than normal folks. My mental diet needs good food. I am aware of my danger triggers which take me off the path.

March 22

PANIC BUTTON

The entire world is in panic mode with the Corona virus. A great opportunity for us in recovery to put love into practice and quell fear. Others are losing their serenity and acting insane. We can rest easy in the eye of the storm and comfort those who are consumed with terror. We ask ourselves, what am I powerless over and what can I control? Worldwide charts of scary numbers are totally out of our control. We can pray for those in affected areas instead of getting a headache and spinning our brains into sleepless nights. What we can do, is be safe, be clean and quit moving around.

My meeting with my Higher Power is the most important hour of the day. I can miss my home group meetings if need be. I seek a spiritual awakening and stay grateful. I don't have any symptoms yet. If I do at some point, I will deal with it when it happens and not agonize over the possibilities. FEAR, Future Events Appearing Real. Are you watching the CNN and Fox media? How many times I have told you, those guys love disaster and thrive on fear? Their job is to scare you witless and they are good at their job. Turn it off please and read something uplifting or spiritual. Substitute love for all your fears.

I remind myself God is not going to give me more than I can handle. This is a golden opportunity to show love for our fellow man. We have a family song, "Everything is going to be alright."

March 23

GOD IS LOVE

My favorite subject is love, you can never get enough of it. My day begins and ends with love. Most of my prayers have love as part of the verse. Love is the answer to my anger and fears. Gratitude and love are in harmony inside the heart and soul for all of us who have chosen this path. Who could ask for anything more?

Divine Love never fails, but is important to know it must be in your fabric, your heart and not just your words. How often we say, "I love you" to get what we want or keep the peace. Where there is fear, love cannot exist. Faith and love are tied together. If you can practice love every day, you will see a drastic change in your life for the better. We have many love opportunities every day if we look for them.

God is not loving but Love itself. There is no situation enough love won't cure. Here is a prayer called "Love" from the *Twelve Step Prayer Book.* "Love is patient; Love is kind. Love is not jealous; it does not put on airs; it is not snobbish. Love is never rude; it is not self seeking; it is not prone to anger; neither does it brood over injuries. Love does not rejoice in what is wrong, but rejoices with the truth. There is no limit to love's forbearance, its truth, its hope, its power to endure."

March 24

LINKAGE

Got someone who you just cannot forgive? Well guess what, you have provided a link stronger than steel. We know resentments are a killer for us. They imprison you like cellmates in the same cell going nowhere. They are always with you in your head. Being right doesn't make your cellmate go away. You are bound to the bad guy with a mental chain, right or wrong. You must let this resentment go free so you can become free again. Release with love was something I learned a few years ago and it works wonders. If you have the willingness to forgive you have a chance. Without it, welcome to a ball and chain.

Let's flip the coin. Forget about resentments and ask yourself who do you want to be linked to? Easy answer. I want to have linkage to my Higher Power. I want Him in my camp to protect me against temptations and negative thinking. Just the opposite of having an enemy as a cell mate. Now I have a powerful friend partnered up with me to form a winning team. As I review my blessings, it is clear God has already filled my basket with gifts to overflowing. This linkage thing can be misery or pure bliss. "Who's in your head?" Ask yourself who has taken up residence in your brain rent free?

We often cannot choose the people we work with. But we can choose who we link up with in our minds and hearts. I choose my Higher Power and have set all my enemies free with love.

March 25

TRANQUILITY

Dangling your bare feet into Walden's Pond conjures up an image of tranquility. Walden's Pond will not make you tranquil unless you already have a tranquil heart. Some folks do a geographic move to find peace and tranquility. They think a tranquil location will improve their mental state. Unfortunately, a new place will not bring the desired change. We have to change ourselves first. I moved around always thinking life would get better with each move. But my alcoholism was increasing. I was getting worse with each drink and wondering why my moves did me no good. Peace, serenity, happiness and tranquility are all inside jobs.

Gratitude is the first feeling of my day, as I thank God for one more day of life. I am still healthy and everyone in my family has been spared from the virus. It is up to us with a grateful, peaceful heart to set the example of tranquility. Others around us are in panic, fearing events not real, only imagined. Panic can be contagious. Our calm attitude and serenity can be contagious. My advice is, if you are not sick, don't move. Trust God and have faith. I am not going anywhere until the storm passes. It is time for reflection and study.

It does my heart good to be able to send out messages of love and hope as God speaks through me. I have food, water and a safe roof over my head. I focus on the peace and tranquility of the moment.

March 26

REVISION

When we reach the turning point in our lives and put down the drink for the last time, our entire life is up for revision. For some reason I thought I would finish the 12 steps and say "done." I soon learned all the steps are up for constant revision. My concept of a Higher Power keeps expanding over time. My readings make it clear if I am really growing a revision of old ideas is required. Recently I misplaced my gratitude list. No problem. I made a new list and was surprised my list went from 44 items to 64. Shows me how much I have grown. This is a good thing.

Emmet Fox warns against having "sacred cows" that block off entire sections needing revision. If you have self-made limitations and say, "I can't stop smoking," or "I can't be around my family." Most of us have some cows out in the pasture. I know I think I can never play a musical instrument or paint a picture. I gave up on these "sacred cows" and have not tried. I have not been willing to give them a test run. If I open my mind, maybe I can open up new horizons I never dreamed were possible. I never imagined not drinking and look at me now.

I can replace "OK" with good. I can replace good with better. I can replace better with best. I don't need to be the master of anything. I will never be perfect. I can undergo constant revision to keep moving upward.

GOD MAKES ME SMILE

Before you ever open your mouth, your face communicates volumes to the outside world. Since this is a program of attraction rather than promotion your forehead to chin is a bill board. If there is a scowl on your face there is a big "off" flag waving folks away. A smile lights up the bill board and says, "I am approachable, I am available." Smiles are free. Smiles send out positive vibes and are usually returned in kind. I live in Thailand, the Land of Smiles. I brought my smile to where it is normal behavior. There are many places a frown is the look of the day. Negative begets negative. No, thank you.

Lucky for me I have no problem smiling all the time. When I was hitting my bottom, I lost my cheerful countenance and was in deep depression. As soon as I found AA and began my recovery my smile returned by the grace of God. When I pray, I smile. When I think of God, I smile. When I look at all the gifts God has bestowed on me, I smile. When I attend a meeting and see all my friends, I smile and laugh. I enjoy the harmony of gratitude, humor, laughter, hugs and smiles every single day. It lights my fire and brings sunshine to my soul. If you have trouble smiling then you can start right now today. Practice smiling until it becomes natural.

I am the happiest man on this planet. The way I show it to the world is by my smile God gave me. Every guy I sponsored was not smiling. Twelve steps later they were grinning from ear to ear.

March 28

FORM A TEAM

Once I dropped the "go it alone" attitude I surrendered. I needed outside help to pull out of the hole I dug for myself. The first person to help me was my sponsor. My home group was right there also as part of my recovery team. Then I learned to get direction from the manager, whom I choose to call my Higher Power. I hooked up with a winning team for the first time in my life. Everybody has different skills and a team effort utilizes the variety of talent to form the best team possible. I am a member of the AA dream team.

So why not have your own personal team? Our family operates like a team even though we don't have uniforms or a mascot. My daughters and I have several projects, including the publishing of *Daily Flight Plan*. We operate like a ball club with everybody in a different role. We are The JAX Team. We have experts in artwork, business, finance, advertising and promotion. When we have a team meeting, it is like a reunion. One member books a car, another finds a house. The JAX Team always stays under one roof. We have a master scheduler doing time management. We have a super shopper to do the logistics. We operate like a well-oiled machine.

Think of the people in your life as a team utilizing the different skills of your grouping. If it is love based and the goals are pure, you most likely have a winner. The secret to success is having equal members who love each other.

EXCITEMENT

"Life is not one damn thing after another, it is the same damn thing over and over," quote by Edna St. Vincent Millay. Drinking every day and expecting a different result but only getting drunk again. We are now on the road to recovery. We can break the cycle. We can get excited about life again. My life is very routine but I don't have a negative view like the quote above. I pray and meditate upon awakening, write a love letter and eat healthy. I go to my AA meeting, take a nap, exercise. read, and relax. Boring? I am excited every day and expect nice surprises in my routine. My life is happy, joyous and free. I have many good friends to see and much to learn yet.

I almost lost my life several times. It is easy to get excited just to wake up to another day of life. I look forward to one more day of good stuff. If you lack excitement in your life you can change by putting a spark into your routine. You don't need to jump out of an airplane for excitement. Helping a new guy "get it" is a thrill. He feels good and I feel good. Looking over your gratitude list is always a shot in the arm. Reviewing all the price- less gifts God has bestowed on me brings a smile to my face and an extra beat in my heart. We all got a life "do over" and this time we can get it right.

Most of us are youngsters at this new life way past our imagination. Why not be as enthusiastic as a child without being childish? Time to have fun, laugh and be happy.

March 30

JUDGING OTHERS

Judging other people is a natural human activity. When we first meet someone, we have an instant opinion based on little information. We see how old they are, how they are dressed, and how they greet you. We have a "friend or foe" gut feeling. Not enough information to be right in our judgment. First impressions are sometimes hard to change. We do form an opinion. We should keep it to ourselves and not act on it, especially in a negative way. Better to see how a person acts and observe their behavior. That's still not a 100% correct sample. We can "know" a person for years and still not be a good judge of their character. Every person is one of God's kids. He or she is our brother or sister. All the rest is a guess.

The flip side is, you are judged rightly or wrongly all the time. Again, not many people really know the real you. All of us are a work in progress. Hopefully we are changing for the better every day. In my working life, I moved 26 times and changed jobs over 40 times. I became an expert on being a "new guy". I had to make a good first impression for those judging me. Being groomed, wearing a smile, being prompt and helpful all was part of my act. The real me was an alcoholic with a selfish heart. I spent a lot of time covering up who I really was.

Being judgmental is not a good idea for us. Resentments are always based on too little information. If we really knew the whole person we resent, we might have empathy rather than disdain.

No

"No" is a complete sentence. One syllable, easy to pronounce. Why do I have such difficulty saying "no"? This blockage of my thinking is one of my most dangerous character defects. There were times my inability to say "no" almost got me killed. Old soldiers preach, "never volunteer for anything." They get old by following this rule. Not me, off into the wild blue yonder in the heart of enemy territory. I could have said, "no". The fear of disappointing others led me to be a "yes" man. Growing up, "yes, sir" was the only correct response. I never told a military boss, "no".

In recovery, for the first time in my life, I learned it was acceptable to say "no". I still hesitate because I feel like I need to explain why I am saying "no". Again, not necessary to add anything else to this complete sentence. Being a people pleaser is one of those character defects hard to reverse. I struggle being agreeable to the point of not being true to myself. When family and friends have a request of me, I have difficulty saying "no". I am such a positive person. "No" is a negative response but one I use more often than ever before.

Being true to oneself should always come before the desires of others. I am still learning. It is not good to compromise myself just to go with the herd. If I listen to my heart, sometimes "no" is the best answer.

April 1

HOW TO MAKE YOURSELF MISERABLE

I am an expert on misery. I can help you get miserable for a long time. First, go someplace where you can be alone and isolate. Get away from those who love you. Take the battery out of your phone. Don't go to any AA meetings. Sit and think just about yourself. If other thoughts enter your mind push them out. Get back to the main topic, you. Next step is to focus on some aches and pains. Think about how the problems will get worse until they kill you. Review the past and all the mistakes in your life. Try to collect all the evidence you can to back up your misery.

Once you get sick and tired of being sick you can reverse the process. You can get out of yourself completely. Push all your selfish demands to the back of your mind. Try to find ways to help others. Find a friend who is miserable like you used to be and cheer him up. Go to an AA meeting every day and get into service. Joke with some friends and take them to lunch. Talk health and happiness to every person you see. Stop thinking about your sore feet. Once we are in a negative spiral it picks up speed until we crash. The upward positive spiral has no limits just heavenly bliss. Gloom and doom are over for me. Thank God.

Be a happy go-giver instead of a miserable go-getter. Misery is optional. The 12 Steps work on my selfish core if I follow directions from my Higher Power. He really wants me to be happy.

OPTIONS

Back in 1974, a former Air Force POW told me, "Every day is good day when there is a door knob on both sides of the door." For five years he had no option. The door was for somebody else. The door was a wall to a POW. Most of us started losing options in our disease. Once we lost the option to not drink, all was lost. We became prisoners. When I heard AA could present some options, I didn't believe it. Going to my first meeting was not an option. I was forced to go by court order. Nothing in my life had any options until I entered AA.

The first day without a drink opened the door I thought was not for me. The gift of sobriety began opening many doors I considered to be locked. Today, I have an array of options. In recovery, I am blessed with options to improve my life. I am not forced to go to AA meetings any more. I have the option to go or not. I want to go. You can't keep me out. If I have a difficult option to consider, I get help. I consult my Higher Power. My friend has two options. Option one, entering Chemo treatment is tiring and causes sickness. Low quality of life but may extend the inevitable a few months. Option two, no Chemo sickness but good quality of life albeit a shorter life span.

There are responsibilities associated with the freedom of options. My options should be God's will not mine. My options should be free of selfish motives.

April 3

WE ARE ALL ONE

Blessed are the merciful. Emmet Fox explains it beautifully, "Because in deed and in truth we are all one, component parts of the living garment of God, you yourself will ultimately receive the same treatment that you mete out to others, you will receive the same merciful help in your own hour of need from those who are farther along the path than you are." A new way of looking at relationships with others for me. Yes, I believe we are all God's kids. I viewed my brother as being over there as a separate entity not as one body. When I condemn my brother, I am condemning myself. When I harm my brother, I am harming myself. When I act negatively toward others it is a lose-lose situation. The whole "body" suffers.

The other key part of the quote is seeking help from those who are on a spiritual path ahead of me. Daily I work on spiritual growth. Maybe I should focus on tapping into the merciful help from those souls further up the mountain than me. I know only a little but I have some resources I can learn from. With this virus covering virtually every country on this planet what more demonstration "we are all one" could you ask for? Praying together, supporting one another we can defeat this virus with no borders.

Holding the thought, we are all one "body" we can all help each other with love. The stronger can pull me up and I can pull those who need my help up at the same time. If the chain is unbroken, we can survive.

April 4

DIG DEEPER

In the AA rooms, I often hear talk of plain raw sobriety. "Happy to be sober." There the story stops. I agree you can't progress without being sober, a requirement for recovery. This is a life long journey without a destination. I need to keep on digging, learning and progressing knowing I will never be perfect. I need to change the old Mike into the new Mike in order to achieve what God wants for me. I need new ideas, new growth and to reach higher into spiritual matters. There is no upper limit to spirituality. It is sad to see so many of my fellows settle for bare bones sobriety. They never change the hateful, resentful person they were before.

In South Africa when they discovered diamonds in the soft yellow clay, some were satisfied with new found wealth and stopped digging. Wiser folks dug deeper into the blue clay and there were 100 times more diamonds with better quality. Same with recovery, the layers go deep and the best is in future spiritual awakenings. They just keep coming slowly but surely. New plateaus can be reached if our faith and willingness to grow is put into action. I seek new teachers, new horizons all the time. I listen for the gems in meetings just like panning for gold. As I look at my extensive gratitude list almost everything on the list is spiritual in nature. I know I am on the right path.

Today I have a thirst for more knowledge and more enlightenment. I know I have only scratched the surface. Dig and dig some more.

April 5

THE TRUTH

We live in an atmosphere of lies and half-truths every day. Most of us have learned what is advertised is not the truth. The best restaurant, best car, best city, is not the best. The military was all lies, the news media lies, politicians lie. We are accepting of all these abortions of truth. It is very hard to separate fact from fiction in our daily lives. Truth just does not have priority in public life. We even turn to super heroes like Spiderman, and Wonder Woman. If only Fantasy Land in Disney World was true life. We need to wake up to the truth.

When I was very young, I could not lie without my ears turning red and cheeks blushing. It took lots of practice but eventually I mastered lies with a straight face. Joining the military was great for me because they are the biggest liars on the planet. "The boys will be home for Christmas," trouble was the year was not specific. It wasn't until I found a spiritual path, truth became a top priority. I had to do a complete inventory to even approach the truth. I do believe God is Truth. To really know truth, I must know God and learn from the Source of Truth. I also learned the truth about life. Caring for others, sobriety, prayer and service was all new stuff. I put the drink down and faced truth in the eye.

Truth never changes. It is. If I turn to my Higher Power for the truth, I get the answer. If I speak the truth, live the truth and seek the truth, I am at peace.

April 6

DESIRE REDUCTION

Many spiritual teachers describe nirvana as a state of self-lessness or absence of all desire. We have overcome the desire for alcohol. We know firsthand the process. I didn't desire the taste of the drink, my desire was oblivion. Stop the world I want off. For a time, I was not part of this world. The Dalai Lama has a great statement on this topic, "There is a drunkenness from the power that we give ourselves over things. This drunkenness leads us to stop controlling our appetites. We want more and still more. Instead of quelling the fire, we reignite it. And we even forget to check whether the fulfillment of our desire is really the one we had wished for."

Satisfactions of desires are so temporary. Take a simple example, ice cream. For five minutes of pure delight my bowl is empty. I feel empty. The gratification from fulfilling my desire is over in a few minutes. On to the next desire. I just consumed a whole week's worth of sugar I need to burn off. It just was not worth fulfilling this desire. I have dropped a number of desires best described as harmful, unnecessary and material in nature. Buddha says enlightenment cannot be reached until the fire of passion and desire are extinguished. Over the last few years, I have noticed my appetite for money, power, prestige and shiny objects are all gone.

My desire is to be helpful to my brothers and sisters. To curb my selfishness. Be happy joyous and free. Desire reduction is simple. Let go and let God.

April 7

LUCK

My Irish heritage is connected to good luck with four leaf clovers. I was brought up on "the luck of the Irish." My family had so many rules about luck you needed a chart. Breaking a mirror will bring seven years of bad luck. If your left hand itches some money was coming your way. All baloney. The Irish do not have the corner on luck as I was taught to believe. I remember hoping the Prize Patrol was going to come and bail me out of my financial woes. God had plans for me and luck had nothing to do with it. I thank God for my good fortune as a result of a spiritual awakening.

Nice surprises, as do tragic events, come and go out of our control. If I stick to the belief every event is supposed to happen, I am on firm ground. I enjoy gambling once in a while. I had runs of good cards and the endorphins started flowing like a drunk. I think it is my skill pulling in the chips. Wrong. I have fun and let the chips fall where they may. I don't want another addiction. In my prayers, I don't ask God for luck. I thank him for the gifts I already have. God will give and take away from me what He wills for my destiny.

The dealers at the gaming tables say "Good luck," but they don't mean it. Better to get the Irish Blessing, "And until we meet again may God hold you in the palm of His hand," and I do mean it.

April 8

THE FIGHTING IS OVER

My entire life was a fight up until my first AA meeting. From birth, I was conscious of war and fighting as part of life. I fought everybody and everything but the biggest enemy was myself. Life was a struggle I thought. Not fighting was something I never considered an option. For us there is no enemy like alcohol. It takes no prisoners. Even with a bullet you can patch up the hole but booze rots the entire body, mind and spirit. At my first meeting I heard "you do not have to fight anybody or anything anymore." The relief I felt from giving up the fight was a spiritual awakening. The air went out of my lungs. I put down my weapons of self-destruction and surrendered.

Someone put our situation like this, "Once we get hooked like a fish in the ocean and dragged out of the sea of alcohol, we end on the floor of the boat. We can flop around and jump back into the ocean. Bad choice. We can fight the program and get beat up by the captain. Best of all, just lie there and stop fighting." After a lifetime of fighting the current, I turned my boat around. I put my fighting oars down and go with the flow. I seek God's will and stop trying to do His job. I stick to my responsibilities and quit managing everybody else's.

The arguments I walk away from make me a winner. All my wars are over. I am unarmed and unafraid. I have lost my craving to do battle.

April 9

HOARDING

Never thought hoarding would be a topic for discussion. This worldwide crisis of COVID-19 has brought out the worst of our fellow earth travelers. I see photos of empty store shelves. I read stories of people standing in line for hours for supplies. Where is the love? No love here, only fear in play with hoarding. Just another word for stealing. If I am stealing from my brother, I am stealing from myself if you believe we are all one body. Taking a year's supply of cleaning products off the shelf so your neighbor has none is totally selfish. If you catch the virus from your neighbor your stock pile becomes useless.

This is an opportunity for sharing of our resources with our brothers and sisters for the greater good. There will be those who don't see the bigger picture. Their selfish behavior is a danger to us all. Some great acts of kindness are coming out to counter balance the harmful ones. Here in Thailand, the food vendors have distributed their entire stock to the growing population of folks out of work. The monks are not allowed out to receive food. Some of the poorest bring what they have to the temples. A culture of giving.

The St. Francis Prayer guides me. "For it is in giving, we receive." I want to meet my Maker with straight eyes, clean hands and an empty shelf.

OH, WHAT A FAMILY

I have seen a lot of fourth step inventories and family issues top the list by far. I have heard many times, "Oh, what a family I have." For some reason, our character defects have family roots. After attending thousands of AA meetings, I never once heard a member talk about what a wonderful family they have. Nobody I know had a *Leave It to Beaver* family. I knew my family was toxic. It took three escape attempts before I got free of the dysfunctional mess. But the damage was done. There are still toxic relationships to this day. There is no family who can hang a shingle outside stating, "Nothing the matter here."

I learned a lot in my fourth step about my past. Most of my character defects had early roots. I wanted love desperately but I had no clue what a relationship should be. I had no role model at all. My relationships were doomed before they ever got started. Being an alcoholic on top of my ignorance equaled disaster. Lucky, I found the rooms of AA to teach me some basics obvious to most folks. My son was the catalyst for the family to gather several times a year. Love and happiness were the order of the day as articulated by my son right up to his last day. He was the epitome of "one day at a time."

Today all of us in my family are grateful for each other. Love abounds and we have reduced resentments to zero. I am now the senior member of my family and lead by example. Love begins here.

April 11

WHO CONTROLS YOUR THOUGHTS?

We often focus on our thought-life and how important it is for our recovery. Before I began my daily routine of prayer and meditation, my thoughts drive me to good use. Before, I never tried to direct my thoughts in any particular direction. My "loose" thoughts were selfishly motivated. My resentments grew, my troubles multiplied and thinking was painful. The only way to stop thinking was to seek oblivion with booze. I would pass out to stop all those voices of doom. The problem was, once I came to from my vacation from thinking, everything was worse. It never occurred to me to pray or control my wild thoughts. A brain without a clutch.

Now in this new life of having a Higher Power in my corner, I can ask for help. Today, I can control my thoughts and program my wellbeing and spiritual condition. I apply a few simple steps of mind control. As soon as I have a negative thought, I can stop it and replace it with a positive thought. It is my choice as to my next thought. No one else controls my thought priorities. I shut off the static of the outside world when I work on my prayer and meditation. This is my time without any outside inputs except what my thoughts are working on. I ask God to direct my thinking and keep my motives pure and stay positive.

The task is to let the language of my heart reach my thought-life. My heart works much better than my brain.

April 12

IT IS ALWAYS NOW

"Stay in the now," we hear so many times but it's hard to do in practice. One of my prayers says it well, "Lord let me do it now for I shall never pass this way again." Meaning this moment is gone forever. The *Big Book* says it best, "That one is God, may you find Him now." If you pray now your prayers will be answered now. If you are in pain, you can focus on God right now this instant. The pain will be secondary. I look to nature for guidance all the time because the messages are right under our noses. Have you ever seen a dog with a watch? A dog stays in the now. A dog doesn't ponder his past or his future.

Our human ego presupposes a sterling future. We have expectations of grandeur and dream on without any guarantees of the future. When reality sabotages our pipe dreams, we get angry and act out. When I buy an airplane ticket, I expect to get my assigned seat. I expect to take off on time, arrive at my destination on time. I have reserved a car. When none of those things really happen, I lose my serenity. I should stay in the now instead and have faith everything is supposed to happen the way it does. Our entire program is built on the philosophy of "one day at a time," so staying in the now is part of our thinking. Putting it into practice is another matter.

I am studying a book called *The Power of Now* by Eckhart Tolle from which I drew my inspiration. It is deep and requires some heavy thought. I recommend you get it now.

April 13

GROWING UP

All those drinking years, no growth took place. No spiritual growth at all, never read a book, never took a class. The years stacked up but maturity stopped decades before. In fact, learning was in reverse as brain cells died with each drink. Instead of growing, I was half dead. I was dying one drink at a time. I rattled off some of my highlights to my boss toward the end of my career and he said, "Yea Mike, great but what have you done lately?" The truth, nothing. At 50 years old on the calendar, I was a teenager in the growth department. When I finally did my inventory, I could see there were huge gaps in my life.

In recovery, life is all about daily growth in body, mind and spirit. Some of the damage to my body is beyond repair but I can take care of the leftovers. For my mind, I have worked hard to catch up to my age by studying every day. In sobriety, I have read hundreds of books compared to none when I was drinking. The spirit was the easiest to repair with the daily routine of prayer and meditation. I know I have miles to go before I sleep but I can see progress very graphically. Each day I try to do a number of things for growth in every area. I have so many years to make up. My guess is I will be 120 years old to break even in knowledge.

Many facets of my life were first learned from joining AA and following the 12 steps. I had no clue on how to sustain a relationship until I put down the drink. Sobriety is a growth industry.

April 14

BENDING OVER FOR THE BOSS

I spent half my life bending over to the desires of parents, bosses and religious leaders. Growing up, I quickly learned the mental torture for non-compliance was not worth the trouble. In my working life, I had to please my boss if I expected to get promoted. The annual report card was a make-or-break deal. I could turn blue if required or jump thru my butt on request. I danced to the tune somebody else picked for me. Amazingly, I did a lot of the right things but for the wrong reasons. It wasn't from my heart. It was self-preservation and selfishness. Down deep, I wanted to cut loose from the pack and go wild.

Those days of bending into a pretzel for other people are over thank God. I am in charge of my daily inventory. All the blame and credit fall on me. These days I ask my Higher Power to try to find God's will for me and go in His direction. No longer do I bend to the will of conventional wisdom or dictates of a boss. A wonderful freedom. I was very fortunate to go against the flow on smoking. You just were not "cool" if you didn't smoke in my younger days but I held out. Today, I see my friends struggle with their smoking addiction and all the associated health issues.

The people and institutions running my life, actions and thought process are all history now. I answer to God and my heart. The result has been harmony, peace and serenity.

April 15

THE FEAR-EGO CONNECTION

The fourth step is the first step we do anything physical, namely put pen to paper. We see our lives in print. The good, the bad and the ugly. When we inventory our fears, it boils down to fear of not getting what we want or losing what we have. The root of both of those fears is our ego. We feel we deserve riches, respect and power. The selfish way of life has thousands of threats to keep us in fear all the time. We can see our actions based on fear were harmful to everybody. We were dishonest to get what we thought we needed. We were angry, which is a form of fear, with ego at the center.

Unfortunately, the ego can never be satisfied. It devours all in its path. Humility and honesty are core requirements for recovery. Those two things are missing in the fear-ego self. It will be impossible to find serenity and peace if the ego self is not brought down to the correct size. Some of the spiritual leaders will argue the ego does not exist, it is an invention of man. I know I was full of fear because I had no faith. My ego-fear self, took me to a very dark bottom. Booze was my medication to combat my fears. Finally, I was properly mangled enough to surrender.

My ego almost killed me. I look back at myself, drowning in sea of alcohol too proud to grab a life preserver. Thank God I was able to reduce my ego-fear connection enough to get rightsized.

April 16

LIFE IS A GRINDSTONE

From *Body, Mind & Spirit*, "Life is a grindstone. But whether it grinds us down or polishes us up depends on us." So true and a good way to look at the grind of daily life. Our attitude can help us get polished or perish. In the military we have a slogan in Latin: "*Illegitimus non carborandum*" which means don't let the bastards grind you down. Sure enough, we had enough bastards to grind you up and spit you out. The point is, every rough grind is an opportunity depending on how we handle it.

In my military history, I had a boss who tried to grind me up and have me kicked out. He was only my boss for 24 hours but he was so angry he booted me out of Laos. Lucky I no longer was under him. I could fight back with correctness. He used illegal means to trash me and it backfired in his face. In my new job, in a different country, I polished the bad situation into a jewel. I got promoted early from the experience and my tormentor was so upset he tried to stop my promotion. Again, it backfired. He retired and I stayed on for 16 more years.

My face has been pushed against the grindstone many times. You can spot my polished head from a mile away. I get shined up every morning.

A BLESSED GATHERING OF SCREW-UPS

Let's take a look at organizations and what makes them work or fail. If I want to join the Oakland A's Baseball Club, I need to be in top physical shape and either hit the ball very well or pitch a 100 mph fastball. If I am better than 95% of other players, I have a shot at making the club. If I want to be a stock broker, I need to have excellent knowledge of the market and a history of success or I will be out of a job. Most organizations have the best people in a particular field of endeavor. How about AA as an organization? You need to be a screw-up to join. We are brothers in our defects rather than our virtues.

On the surface it looks like AA can't possibly be successful. It has proven itself to be the road to recovery for millions of suffering screw-ups. It is backwards from the traditional organization. Basically we are spiritually centered, finding a Higher Power and recovering from a seemingly hopeless condition. We are not about making a profit. We are not about fame. We are not competing with any other entity. We have no outside interests past staying sober and helping other alcoholics. Singleness of purpose.

We are truly blessed to be in this gathering of former screw-ups, getting better one day at a time. New screw-ups keep us alive and growing. Best organization I ever joined.

April 18

A New Dimension

A reading about a "new dimension" brought to mind the many new levels of spiritual progress as a result of recovery. In my inventory, I look at where I was before I finally surrendered. I was about 5% alive 0% useful. My health had me at death's door, liver way off the chart, overweight and high blood pressure. My spiritual life was non-existent. Totally broke and unemployable. When I think about where I started, I thank God I am even alive to tell the story. The first big dimension was the relief from the obsession to drink. Next dimension was happiness. I thought happiness would never happen for me and I didn't deserve any joy. Then came the 12 Steps.

Each Step is a dimension in itself. Each Step, when fully realized, was a new spiritual awakening. Doing Step 4 and 5 made the earth move under my feet. It was a turning point from being an attendee to a fully vested member of AA on the road to long term sobriety. Then the realization helping others and being of service was as rewarding as finding diamonds under my pillow. The wonderful dimension of sponsoring other guys and see them "get it". As the years go by, the growth keeps taking me to new plateaus of spiritual awakenings. The biggest dimension of all was finding a Higher Power in my camp every day. I am not alone anymore.

From 5% alive, today I am at 100%. I know new dimensions await me as long as I keep the faith and do what I know works.

April 19

LIFE IS A BUFFET

Great personal story from Emmet Fox on his first trip to America. He stopped in a busy restaurant and selected a table and sat down. He waited quite a long time and he saw everyone around him eating and enjoying their dinner. He felt left out until it finally dawned on him it was a buffet. Fox likens his experience to the way the universe is run. You have to claim your nourishment. If you wait for what you want to come to you it might never happen. Life is like a buffet in many ways as we make selections to nourish our body, minds and spirit. I always seemed to pick the wrong things for my plate.

Today I can carefully select the healthiest food for my body and control the portions. For my mind, I can choose what I read, watch and listen to. I have eliminated junk food. I have eliminated stuff to rot my brain and steal time from my day. For my spirit, my buffet of readings and prayers kept me in top spiritual condition for a long time. The diet is working. In the past, my picker was broken. I made bad choices at the buffet table. I picked the wrong career path for half my adult life. I stopped at the bar too many times before making choices. The results were predictable.

The difference today is, I ask for help in my selections of life's buffet. My Higher Power pokes me in the ribs when I reach for the wrong things.

April 20

YOU ARE MY BROTHER

We are all God's kids. I truly believe this and must, by conscience, treat every person as my brother or sister. Not in a theoretical sense but in actuality. I must accept this relationship in my heart not just in verbiage. My spiritual readings tell me if I have difficulty with my brother then I need to make peace quickly and resolve the problem. Am I my brother's keeper? Absolutely. I am responsible to my human family to support my relatives in any way possible. Being in service to my human family is basic to do my part in the community of man. When you remove anger, resentments, greed, fear what you have left is love. If I am angry with my brother, I will never know serenity.

The basic prayer Our Father makes it clear. We all have the same loving Father, thus we are brothers by definition. We are separated by language, location, politics, color and economic wellbeing. We are still brothers and sisters but fear has put up walls and borders. Greed has hoarded food away from our brothers who are starving to death. We should be loading a truck with our abundance and driving across the border. We could lovingly donate necessities to a family member. Living in an international community opens my heart to hug a Russian and take an Iranian out to dinner. Some mental borders had to be broken down in my own mind.

Thinking of everyone as my brother needs to be in my heart, not just in rhetoric. I vow to meet every person who crosses my path with a smile and put love into my every action. You are my brother.

April 21

DISCIPLINE OF THOUGHT AND SPEECH

I have good inventory sessions with my conscience. I still need to clean my brain and my manner of speech. My spiritual teacher tells me if I commit murder in my imagination, I am guilty of sin by harboring such thoughts. Sometimes I imagine my enemies having an accident. I need to control such wanderings of my thought process. My time would be more spiritual if I would think of ways to break the negative pattern of my thinking. I just read about a motor-cyclist who died by losing control of his machine giving somebody the finger. I often give the finger mentally. I need to stop before I crash in some other way.

My home group is an all-male affair most mornings. The language gets salty, to say the least. If the "f" word was elim-inated there would be an extra 10 minutes for someone else to share. I have realized, I have an off switch to my speech. If I am upset with the IRS, I tend to curse out the faceless bastards making my life miserable. It says more about me and my spiritual condition than it does about some automated response from a government computer. I need to remember how I speak. It shows the world my true character. Discipline of speech is important and keeping my big mouth shut is always a good option.

My point is, discipline and thoughtfulness are key to long term serenity. Spicing my speech with anger is hurtful to me and others. My thinking needs good orderly direction.

April 22

SHINE YOUR LIGHT

"Let your light so shine before men, that they may see your good works, and glorify your Father which is in heaven." (Matthew 5:16) The state of your spiritual condition shows in what you radiate in your outer condition. One writer says, "Your face shouts more about what is in your heart than your words." If loving kindness resides in my heart, the light will shine. Emmet Fox puts it this way, "The soul that is built upon prayer cannot be hidden, it shines out brightly through the life that it lives." We all know people who radiate goodness. My life has been blessed by close association with a number of shining souls.

The message is clear, living a spiritually centered life will attract others to your light. Before my recovery, my light was out. My appearance shouted, "Leave me alone, don't bother me." A long process of turning on my light took years after living in darkness for decades. The 12 Steps were just a start. The spiritual awakening, as a result of doing all the Steps, flipped the switch to on. Sure enough, my light attracted others to ask for help. Eventually their light was shining also.

My attitude of gratitude, love, and caring turns on my green "available" light. From the St. Francis Prayer, "that where there are shadows, I may bring light."

April 23

HOUSE CLEANING

Just think about never cleaning your house for 30 years. The house I'm referring to is your inventory. It is our mess. Only we can clean it up with help from a Higher Power and a sponsor we trust. There may be some crimes hidden in the junk pile and some debts needing payment. A clean house is allowing open loving relationships with honesty. No ugly baggage to clutter up the picture. A clean house makes you feel good about yourself. The freedom coming from dumping out all the past garbage has to be experienced to understand how weightless a person can feel. It is like flying without wings.

I had some stuff 50 years old. It does not go away. It just sits in your soul and rots. It needs to come out of the vault and be defrosted. If you really want to totally clean house, like the steps ask for, it must be addressed 100%. My suggestion is get started. Drop the bag today, not tomorrow. Start in one room, harms to others for example. Work your way to the next room, such as fears. Save the biggest room for last, resentments. Write an outline of your life all the way up to the present. Try to recall the first candy you stole from the super market at six years old. Go from there.

The trick is to keep your house clean once you have done a thorough scrub and polish. Only you can drop the rock you have been carrying around in your heart.

April 24

FEAR MANAGEMENT

Today happiness management is my problem. I am so happy it is hard to absorb it all. So many gifts. The biggest decision I have to make is which is better, which is best. Before happiness management, came fear management. Once I passed the course, I could move on to being happy joyous and free. My entire life up until I found the rooms of AA was fear based. There were so many things wrong in my life, fear was the result. We learn the hard way, faith trumps fear 100% of the time. I joined a fear group, the military. I played a small part in a possible nuclear war working on B-52's headed for Russia. Total fear and terror.

Then I entered the world of combat, spinning the roulette wheel of death every day. Several glasses of courage every night helped. I had a sobering experience of intense fear my life was over in a combat situation. I knew if taken prisoner booze will no longer be available. Fear of detoxing in captivity motivated me into drastic action. My fear management went straight to prayer. It worked miracles then as it does today. Prayer solidifies my faith in God. I admit my powerlessness in my plea for help. I cannot say I am fearless today but now I know how to manage my fears.

Today I know I am not alone. Through prayer, I am connected with my Higher Power who will be in charge of all my fears. I am convinced everything is supposed to happen in God's time.

April 25

COME FLY WITH ME

If you fly with me, I guarantee a safe pleasurable journey. No baggage to carry and no long lines at the airport. Just because we are all locked down until the virus is contained doesn't mean we cannot fly with the angels spiritually. To fly with me there is no negativity, no fears allowed to invite dark stormy weather. Take out your gratitude list and read each item. The boost from a grateful heart will give you enough lift for the flight.

This lock down time can be a pain or an opportunity. April is inventory month. A coincidence? A good time for self-improvement and self-examination. Time for all kinds of house cleaning. Time to read some good books to fly you out of the four walls at home. I am in Indiana right now rescuing a wrongly accused man from the death penalty. The book I am reading took me there. I will be home for dinner in warm cozy Thailand. Every day I see folks from six different time zones on my Zoom meetings. We are blessed by many channels of communication.

We have many ways to fly mentally and spiritually. Our mobility has closed one door but other doors are open to be free from bondage. We can reach out all across the globe with love and friendship.

Forgiveness in Advance

In AA the most important things are quite simple and obvious. We all know firsthand resentments are the number one killer for us alcoholics. What is the Rx for curing resentments? Forgiveness, carefully spelled out in our 11th Step Prayer. If you cannot forgive the resentments, they will haunt you. If you cannot forgive, you are burning the bridge you need to cross. Hanging on to resentments rots the soul. Serenity is impossible. Once you learn to forgive, the freedom you feel will make you weightless. You carry the person you resent around in your head rent free.

If we want to be free of resentments, forgiveness is the solution, why not practice forgiveness ahead of time? Get yourself into a forgiving mindset before an incident happens requiring forgiveness. This means I forgive you even before I meet you and there is any interaction. If I really believe in acceptance then I know I must accept my brothers as they are, not as I would have them be. Some might strike out at me, at least verbally, but I need not engage. I can step sideways and let any aggression pass on by and not push back. I am trying to change and give up ground in the name of peace.

Today I can spot events or certain folks who are dangerous to my serenity. If I mix it up with them, I will need to practice forgiveness later on. Why not skip a forgiveness opportunity by being absent?

April 27

DEATH IS NOT THE END

My son, Mike passed away three years ago from Lou Gehrig's disease. I hear his laugh and see his face every morning in my first hour of prayer and meditation. His loving spirit lives in my heart even though I can't hug him anymore. His death was not a surprise. We had six years to prepare for the inevitable. The Dalai Lama has much to say about death. Here is just one quote, "If you are mindful of death, it will not come as a surprise—you will not be anxious. You will feel that death is merely like changing your clothes. Consequently, at that point you will be able to maintain your calmness of mind."

My son must have channeled the Dalai Lama because he was the world's calmest person when he passed. His love and character live on with his family and the entire community of Mystic, CT. The lessons he taught us live on and grow. Three members of my home group have passed recently. We have an extensive webpage dedicated to our departed brothers. I hope and pray the messages of hope and love I have received are passed on 200 years from now to a newly recovering alcoholic.

I truly believe our good works will live on long after our bodies quit. I can only leave a spiritual message since I will only be a spirit after the final curtain. A new exciting dimension is yet to come.

April 28

IT IS EITHER LOVE OR FEAR

My spiritual teacher knocked me over with this one. Human feelings boil down to either love or fear. Period. I tried to come up with an exception but failed. What about anger? It is fear in disguise. Hatred, ego, jealousy, aggression, criticism and arrogance are all rooted in fear. Love based feelings are easier to see. Prayer, service, kindness, giving, smiles and encouragement are clearly love based. Passion can be full of hatred or full of love depending on how you "feel". I always tell my wife she cooks with love thus every meal is wonderful. Love is always constructive. Fear is always destructive.

Love is the answer. In recovery, my life is love centered. My day begins and ends in love. Prayer upon awakening and a "thank you God for another wonderful day," when I sleep. My gratitude list fuels my attitude with love and happiness all day long. In the old days, it was just the opposite, fear upon awakening and chaos all day. One of the members tagged me as love bug. Another guy said if I am happy all the time, I am a sick puppy. I can live with my sickness no problem. I know God loves me and prayer is how I thank Him.

Which mindset, either the one of fear or one of love is entirely up to us. We can choose. I want to be constructive for the rest of my days.

Spiritual Bank Account

My first AA meeting the secretary talked about a "spiritual bank account." I have never forgotten her explanation. I learned you can open your spiritual account immediately and make a deposit with prayer for starters. When you go to meetings, do the steps, get in service, you make deposits to your spiritual bank account. There is no upward ceiling to how much you can deposit into your account. The basic idea is to have lots of "cash" on hand. You can write a check to handle any emergency without going broke, as in getting drunk again.

You never know what life might dish out at any given time. The unexpected death of a loved one. You lose your job. A shock to the system often brings thoughts of a drink. If your spiritual bank account is full up you can write a check and stay sober no matter what. In Buddhist terms we call this "making merit". The idea is the same. Keeping your spiritual wellbeing in top shape when things are going well. This will insure you can weather any storm. My connection with my Higher Power gave me the faith to accept a bumpy ride down the road of life.

In the past, I would not pray until my fat was in the fire. I prayed only in emergencies. Bad idea. I try to max out my spiritual bank account the same way I maxed out my credit cards.

TRANSFER OF POWER

In an aircraft with a stick, the pilot in command shakes the stick as he says, "I've got the aircraft." This signals the other pilot to take his hands off the controls. Every morning my Higher Power says "I've got it." The power needs to go to the one most qualified to run my life, God. Since I cannot see my pilot in command, I tend to put my grimy mitts on the stick. I transfer the power back to myself. Soon we are in heavy turbulence and thunder storms. I stall out and get myself into a tailspin. Then I look to the Chief Pilot to shake the stick and stop the dive before I crash and burn.

"May I do Thy will always." I say every day in my 3rd Step Prayer. The "always" part is where I stumble on occasion. Forgive me, but I spent a good part of my life not sharing stick time with another pilot. Old habits come back and I think I need to take control of the situation. I see some folks forget. Once they start to feel better and improve their life's circumstances, they say, "OK God and fellowship, I will take it from here." I have never seen a successful "graduation." I know I must seek God's will for me daily.

I can say the words of my prayers easily but I have to accept the words in my heart. Transferring power over to my Higher Power is the ultimate goal of my morning prayer and meditation.

May 1

HEALING

Seven years ago, I had a fall in front of my building. It came close to killing me. I slipped on a wet ramp and hit my back on a sharp point of a stair. The blunt force cracked a rib which punctured and collapsed a lung. Ten level pain got worse during a clumsy X-ray session. The doctor sent me home to die. The real problem was a severed bowel leaking poison into my body. I was toughing it out for a few days until finally I surrendered to a major hospital. My surgeon met the ambulance and operated immediately. He saved my life in the nick of time.

A side effect of my new bowel equipment was constant discomfort. I was prepared to live with it for the rest of my life. Just recently I have been blessed with a breakthrough. The condition is healed. First hand, I know the body keeps trying to repair itself. Patience is required. The older you are, the longer it takes. Emmet Fox discusses healing extensively. His point always amounts to being positive. Don't focus on your malady and cultivate more pain. Think of God and the problem will disappear according to Fox. I can verify what he taught me.

A huge lesson I learned. You are in charge of your medical team. Doctors are human beings. One doctor almost killed me, another saved me. Spiritual healing through prayers works.

May 2

FOCUS THE SINGLE EYE

If you want to cross a river by walking on a log, the trick is to focus on the goal ahead. Don't look down. You will get wet if you do. All great achievers testify their success came from a sharp focus on the objective and tenacity. Most people who have reached the summit of whatever mountain they had to climb had to overcome some difficulties. For us, it is simple, we have but one single purpose. Stay sober and help others stay sober. We focus on the goal. We maintain our spiritual condition in the best shape possible. We keep our focus sharp.

Many religions and spiritual teachings talk about the "single eye". The idea is to see the objective clearly and not be diverted to outside interests. "Man cannot serve God and mammon at the same time." (Matthew 6:24) Clearly the message is to seek God and be in His grace. Reject the attraction to material objects. The diamond cutter has a single eye piece to do the delicate work of shaping a diamond correctly. When you thread a needle, you close one eye to focus correctly. The "single eye" gets the proper attention to the task. Whatever you steadfastly direct your attention to, will come into your life.

I am certain if the Glory of God comes first with me, His will runs my life. I will be filled with light and happiness.

BREAKING THE RULES

Alcoholics don't follow rules well. Lucky our AA founders gave us only "suggestions". My favorite saying from the Dalai Lama, "Learn the rules so you know how to break them properly." At fourteen years old I attended the seminary to be a priest. They had a rule, if you leave the facility you cannot return. I ventured into the city to see a movie. I got caught. I was thrown out of the seminary. For sure, I would have become an alcoholic priest. I broke rules in the Air Force and scammed my way into pilot training. I did become a pilot. This success almost killed me.

Some good fortune comes from rule breaking. Somebody has to push the envelope. Chuck Yeager broke the sound barrier when engineers thought the aircraft would come apart. One myth was debunked and Chuck became a hero. Lucky for us in AA there are no "rules" but some truisms are hard and fast. There is an unwritten rule, "no relationships in your first year of sobriety". Mr. Rule Breaker crossed the time line. It smacked me in the face when a relationship went south. I had no credits in my spiritual bank account. The slip scared me to the core. I did all 12 Steps quickly then.

I still like to challenge rules. I choose my battles more carefully. One simple rule remains true in every case, "Don't take the first drink and you won't get drunk." I do follow this truism.

May 4

CONSTANT TREATMENT

All of us on the road to recovery realize we need to treat our disease. Most us do not use the term "recovered". My recovery will never be finished. My condition needs constant treatment. My treatment program works for me. It may not do the job for someone else. Everything we do for our body, mind and spirit is a treatment. Some treatments heal. Others make the condition worse. In the case of medicine, I have learned to be cautious. If the doctor says this pill will stop swelling there is a good chance my swelling will get worse. My chemistry is strange. I am not normal at anything.

I use a daily "treatment" of good literature and block out media negative inputs. For my body, I eat healthy balanced food in proper portions. My exercise is a treatment in flexibility. I know for my alcoholism, I am only given a daily reprieve based on my spiritual condition. After decades of self-destruction, it will take decades of healing. My treatment program is not only constant, it is ever increasing. I search for new ideas and new methods of "treatment". I must stay vigilant for negative treatment to stop the healing process.

My thought-life drives the treatment in all aspects of my life. It is in my best interests to stay positive. I seek God's help to get better each day. I am in charge of my treatment plan.

TIME IS MY FRIEND

Time either flies or drags depending on your attitude. One of my readings talks about, "Time is the only cash you have so spend it wisely." For some, time is the enemy, always late for appointments and work. I have the attitude time is my friend. Time is on my gratitude list. God has given me enough sober time to do the 12 Steps many times over. Time to make amends to the best of my ability. My Higher Power has given me the time and tools to make peace with everyone who would accept my love.

I manage my time as if it was gold. I try to eliminate time wasters like watching news I have no control over. Every morning there is a prayer I say called Take Time. "Take time to think, it is the source of power. Take time to play it is the secret of perpetual youth. Take time to read it is the fountain of wisdom. Take time to pray, it is the greatest power on earth. Take time to be friendly, it is the road to happiness. Take time to laugh, it is the music of the soul. Take time to give, it is too short a day to be selfish. Take time to do charity, it is the key to Heaven."

I know time is my friend because all my emotional, spiritual and physical wounds have disappeared. I try to live in God's time and thank Him for every minute.

OLD ME, NEW ME

I thank God every day for transforming the old me into the new me. The Steps have changed me. I knew I needed a complete make over. My daily morning meeting with my Higher Power never happened with the old me. In the morning session I read my gratitude list. The old me had no list. Not one of the 64 items on my list would go on a list written by the old me. Yes, I experienced a life do-over with drastic changes of character. The old me was aggressive, controlling, and ego driven. Today, the new me aspires to be a fairly quiet sober member of the AA fellowship.

As I review my character defects, it seems many are squashed and have disappeared. I found some defects still inside my lock box. They may be dormant. Those hidden defects raise their ugly head if the situation arises to re-open the defects box. I avoid possible situations where my known vulnerabilities have a chance to resurface. If I am around my wartime buddies the stories begin to flow. If I open my yap, I will have a better story. Today my old buddies find me rather boring. "What happened to you Mike?" Got sober and had my ego reduced. Thank God.

I guess some defects I have are in my blood and bone marrow. All of us would be pretty bland without some real fun flaws for all to enjoy.

May 7

BE GOOD TO YOURSELF

I have a good friend who always says goodbye with the message, "Be good to yourself." I need to hear and practice his advice. You are told aboard every aircraft flight, "Put on your own oxygen mask first before you try to help others put on theirs." If you don't take care of your own needs first, eventually you will be out of service to everybody including yourself. I was also a workaholic. My mind was work focused only and my spiritual life was non-existent. Today I take care of my body with a balanced diet and my mind with good inputs. If I take care of my spiritual well-being, everything else will follow.

In Thailand, if there is a sickness in the family, a worker will walk off the job and deal with family first. In my culture, you might get fired if you just walk away from your job to care for family. I will leave it up to you which is the best route to take. I know I must put my spiritual condition first and foremost. If I lose my sobriety all else is lost. I take time to exercise every day. I just do it. I ask myself the question. "Mike, you want to live a little longer or do you want to die?" I have dozens of choices every day. I try to do what is best for my body, mind and spirit. I may have to be a bit selfish from time to time.

If my goal is to help others, I can't help anyone if I am grounded for repairs. A newcomer is not going to ask me for help if I look sickly and tired. Healthy sobriety is attractive.

RELATIONSHIPS 101

I guess I was behind the door when they gave the course on relationships. When I finally got some help with a class on relationships it pointed out my relationships had one common factor, me. Since it was impossible to blame all the other folks the problem was clearly mine. Then in recovery I learned all my relationships were based on my selfishness. A big part of recovery was the change from a "taker" into a "giver". Before I woke up to reality, I would only enter into a relationship if I had something to gain. Sooner or later the giver will stop giving. They get tired of being used and manipulated.

I learned to be a loving person thinking of others. Just like my daily prayer says, "To be just as enthusiastic about the success of others as I am about my own." The idea is to enter into relationships with the mindset of "what can I give to this relationship?" instead of "What can I get from it?" I see in my own culture 50-50 type relationships. I prefer to enter into relationships with another "giver". When two "givers" join up both give 100%. The love math comes out to be a 200% loving relationship.

A blessing of this program is the joy of meaningful relationships. First, I had to love myself in order for love to flow both ways.

May 9

HAIL THE CONQUEROR

"Though he should conquer a thousand men in the battlefield a thousand times, yet he, indeed, who would conquer himself is the noblest victor." Quote from Buddha. This phrase on the opening page of a book on Buddhist teaching spoke volumes to me in my early sobriety. In my distorted image of myself, I was a warrior and a conqueror of sorts. I bought into the graphics of power, swords, and flaming guns. All hype to fit the role of winning battles. Was I not a Dragon or a Raven as my title? All false persona. When they took away my aircraft and my gun, I had only one enemy to face. Myself.

In Laos, we fought to control the Plain of Jars in the center of the country. Having pushed the enemy back for a time we were able to land in the battlefield for the first time. My crew chief was already in place with fuel when I landed. He shouted, "Hail the conqueror." Who had I liberated? No one. A few months later, the Plain of Jars was lost again and belongs to the opposition to this day. Being a conqueror was an illusion. I was and am, powerless. The only person I can conquer is myself. There will be no parade for the conquest. My Higher Power knows and I know, the battle has been won.

Doing the 12 Steps repeatedly has defeated the enemy within me. Faith and love have overwhelmed fear and resentment. Every day of sobriety is a victorious day.

May 10

TROUBLE INTO HARMONY

Whenever I see the word "harmony" I flash back to 1982 and the song *Ebony and Ivory* by Paul McCartney and Stevie Wonder. The first line, "Ebony and ivory live together in perfect harmony" makes clear reference to black and white people living in harmony. In America, we have come a long way from the racially troubled times of the 60's. Riots in Watts and Oakland, the assassination of Martin Luther King are part of our history. The world does get better in my view. It has been 75 years since the last World War. I pray we learn from today's world-wide virus and make our planet safer. We need to find harmony regardless of national interests and politics.

Emmet Fox stresses prayer will change things and prayer works. In troubled times if you act *as if* there was harmony along with prayer, the trouble will disappear. To struggle with the trouble makes it worse by agitating the situation. If a trouble maker approaches a loving attitude and a cheerful smile it will disarm the hostile person. I am still working on this one. I tend to return a scowl with a scowl instead of a harmonious look. Fox promises, "The fact is that seeing the Presence of God where the trouble seems to be does not merely give us courage to meet the trouble; it changes the trouble into harmony."

The Dalai Lama agrees, "And it seems to me that nowadays the spirit of harmony is increasing, that our desire to live together calmly is growing stronger and stronger."

May 11

MENTAL ASSENT

When we pray, we are giving mental assent to communication with our Higher Power. This is a good thing. We become what we think, read, listen to and watch. If you watch the news, you are saying, "Go ahead, I am listening." What book you pick up and read, you are giving carte blanch for the contents of the book to work in your thoughts. It also applies to resentments. If you allow your thoughts to dwell on a person who has harmed you, then you have approved entry into your thoughts. For good or harm, nothing enters your thought process without your consent.

The first hour of prayer and meditation is so important to give your brain a spiritual awakening of your choice. Don't let CNN start your brain working. They have nothing good to say. If you read and watch garbage then junk will enter your thought life. No action happens without a thought coming first. The key is assent to truth and love for brain food. In your personal Secret Place, you can communicate with your Higher Power who possesses all Intelligence and Truth. Block out static and non-productive thinking. Prayer and meditation will get you to where you should be.

I recently left two of my friends shouting at each other on the street. I choose not give assent to the anger or worse, pick one side over the other. I voted with my feet by not participating in the fray.

REGENERATION

"Regeneration means building a new mentality; that is, creating a new soul in place of your present one." Quote from Emmet Fox. My defeat at the result of my drinking is my greatest victory. It opened my mind to doing a complete change in my spiritual life. I must change for the better and it will not happen overnight. It took 30 years of wrong thinking and wrong actions to hit my total defeat. Thirty years of prayer and meditation is a decent start to remaking my soul. I know I must change in my heart and soul in order to radiate peace and harmony. The vibes I put out need to come from within. I need to be the real deal if I am going to help others.

I am truly grateful for all the gifts God has bestowed on me. I am a happy person. Everyone knows I am super happy without me thinking about it or faking happiness. Hopefully, my smile says "I am approachable, I am available to you." Page 164 from the *Big Book*, "You cannot transmit something you haven't got." Whatever is in your heart and soul is the real you. My insides had a major regeneration, not near finished. Much different than the loud, egotistical idiot at the bar holding court.

I can read great things. Only when I put the good thoughts into solid action does it filter down from my head. From there it enters my heart for a permanent change and regeneration.

May 13

LANGUAGE OF THE HEART

A good friend, of 55 years, explained to me what it was like to be alone on the open ocean for a month. He said the sailor's prayer every day, "Dear God, be good to me. The sea is so wide, and my boat is so small." Since there was no one to talk to, he would stop verbalizing in his head after a few days of quiet meditation. He was on "watch" all day having cat naps for rest. Instead of thinking in English, he thought in concepts, feelings and images. I suggested to him this was a spiritual experience. "Absolutely," he said. "Going under the boat alone in the open ocean for repairs was a spiritual experience," he reported. "Just me, God and prayer."

This story gets close to what is best described as language of the heart. It is a language different than the language of the brain or the committee of voices we hear all the time. Many spiritual teachers advise, "Listen to your heart." I know my brain is damaged but my heart is good. I must let my heart trump my brain for the best results. Not always an easy task when my brain has a loud argument in progress. First step is quiet, second step is prayer to tap into my Higher Power. He never sends me a text or email. His message always comes in the language of the heart. In order to do the translation, my mind needs to be quiet, positive and at peace.

You need not be on the open ocean alone for a month to learn the language of the heart. The more you use this language the more fluent you will become. Multiple spiritual messages will come through this channel.

May 14

THE OTHER SIDE

A major fear for many is the fear of dying. I have come close to dying so many times, I should be dead. The fear is long gone. First of all, God picks your check out time. Why try to outguess God and fear the future? God will approve your departure if and when He is ready. God has brought me from the brink many times. I have deep faith when the time is right it will happen at God's speed, not mine. Most of us have no idea how much time we have. I am prepared, my family knows what to do. I know one bad fall and it may be lights out in a heartbeat. Just fine with me.

There was a time I did fear death because my life had many loose ends. I had kids to raise, debts to be paid, wreckage needing attention, on and on. I feared death because I knew I was not ready to face God with clean hands and straight eyes. My departure resume was horrible. I was definitely not ready for any afterlife. Today I am not ashamed to transition from this life to the next. The God of my understanding did so well for me in this life. I know the same God is there for me on the other side. What's to fear?

Afraid of hell? My spiritual advisor tells me "hell" is unfulfilled desires and insatiable cravings. I know alcohol gave me a thirst impossible to quench. I have already been to "hell" thank you. I'm not going back.

May 15

I WANT TO BE ALONE

I love my alone time. I have so many things needing attention without anybody else being involved. There is a world of difference between being lonely and being alone. All of us have known the loneliness of our disease. We know the pain of being cut off from all other human beings, stuck with the person we hate the most...ourselves. From the first meeting of AA, I have never been lonely again. I can be alone when I choose solitude and be with family and friends at the right times. It is one kind of "hell" when you want to be alone but cannot because of the situation. For example, being in a drunk tank with 20 gang bangers.

When I am alone, I am with a good friend. I need to be alone in my prayer and meditation to connect with my Higher Power. My favorite hour of the day is the first hour upon awakening. Maybe it is sign of old age but I crave quiet and peace. I remember the days of constant noise, loud music and lots of people around. No more, thank you God. AA conventions are a challenge for me. I love to renew old friendships and quietly sneak out and go home. I have found if I am good company alone, I can be good company with others. Finding the right balance between the two is my challenge.

I think since our bodies need sleep, our minds and hearts need solitude to be fully loving and attentive. Our friends and family deserve the best from us.

May 16

WORLD PEACE

Years ago, I saw a bumper sticker, "Visualize Whirled Peas". Either you could view the sticker as a joke or a mockery of world peace. It is true you must visualize something before it can become reality. I visualize world peace and pray the human race can reach such a state. I practice personal peace, then peace with my Higher Power and my family. I spread the love I have in my heart to every living creature I meet. In my situation, I meet with people from different countries. Some from countries who were at war with my country in the past. My friends don't discuss religion, politics and war. We meet in love and peace. We work on self-improvement to be an asset to our community and give of ourselves.

This Corona virus is a worldwide problem giving humanity an opportunity to find a worldwide solution. Placing blame on one country is negative energy wasted. This virus proves the borders on the map are meaningless. The power of God is also available without borders. Once the antidote is discovered, the challenge will be worldwide distribution. The best solution should be for all, not just the privileged or for profit. Can you visualize this as an opportunity for world peace?

When this virus passes, it will be a different world. As individuals, we are limited but we can connect with One who has all power. Loving kindness can heal our planet and bring us closer to world peace.

YOUR SCOPE

From my spiritual reading, "We ask not any soul to perform beyond its scope." I hope and pray all of you find a scope fitting your talents and desires. It wasn't until I got on the road to recovery did I discover almost my entire time in the military I was way out of my scope and talents. I was undisciplined, rebellious and wild. Lucky, I had many different jobs during those crazy years. One highlighted my talents and desires, an assignment as a teacher. It was my happiest time in uniform. In retirement I did part time teaching for two universities. I was in heaven. If I could do my life over again, I would be a teacher. A sober one, God willing.

Forcing others to work out of their scope is a special sin. In some families the children have their life's work chosen for them. No freedom to choose their desired path. I tried to steer my kids toward education and noble professions. I had the good sense to let them choose their own path. They turned out just fine. Part of the reading is about not being forced to do something you are not capable of doing. It has happened to me many times in my life and I drank over it. Most of us are in a position of freedom to choose our own individual scope. We can walk away from a job not in our scope and pray for one that is.

Today my only job in life is to carry the message of hope to those who still suffer. I love my job. I can do it with some real-life experiences and a deep desire to help others.

FOLLOW YOUR BLISS

We focus too much on our character defects and the negative side of our inventory. Yes, our past must be dealt with but sometimes we have a good side to our past we overlooked. God created all of us to be beautiful people and our job in recovery is to let the real you emerge out of the wreckage. It is a good idea to review your assets and talents. Some talents may have been buried in the blurred years of our disease. There are probably some talents in your kit bag you don't even know about. All of us carry around riches never to be discovered if we don't seek them.

A big step in finding your talents is to remove the limitations. If you say you can't do something then, by God, you can't. If you limit yourself, only you can remove self-imposed barriers. Disregard people who put you down and throw cold water on your dreams. My first-grade teacher would listen to the chorus and come by and say, "Michael you don't have to sing." I was crushed and embarrassed. Then in college I took creative writing because I thought someday, I would be a writer. My instructor wrote on my paper, "You are foggier than London." I quit writing and gave up my dream. Of course, being an alcoholic, all my dreams went up in smoke anyway. I have dusted off this old dream and some professionals think I am a writer of sorts, albeit a novice.

I follow my bliss and write to all of you and hit a cord occasionally with some. I have learned to ask God to guide me toward the talents He has given me.

May 19

THE IMMUNE SYSTEM

We have been told, in our literature, nothing works better than helping another alcoholic to insure immunity from drinking. Our amazing bodies have several immune systems to keep us alive and operating disease free. The God given design of our body does all sorts of activity to preserve life. Our bodies can take a lot of damage and disease and keep on ticking. Our internal immune system is multi-layered to protect us against pathogens like a virus. There are the innate and the adaptive system. The memory function of the adaptive immune system is truly a marvel. It remembers a previous attack and can stop a repeat occurrence. If you had dengue fever once you will not get it again. However, there four different types of dengue.

My point in discussing the immune system is pass on the words of wisdom from Eckhart Tolle the author of *The Power of Now*. He has a dissertation on strengthening the immune system. "The more consciousness you bring into the body, the stronger the immune system becomes. It is also a potent form of self-healing. When you inhabit your body, it will be hard for unwanted guests to enter." He goes on to discuss self-healing meditation and Emmet Fox talks extensively on the same theme. The mind can control much of how the body operates both in a positive or a negative way. It is up to us to bring harmony to body, mind and spirit.

I have put this to the test as soon as symptoms appear. I flood my body with consciousness. I have not had a cold or the flu in 30 years. A heavy dose of positive, spiritual thinking has done wonders for me.

YOUR PLAN GOD'S PLAN

A few of my spiritual readings focus on God's plan for all of us. There is an old joke going around if you want God to laugh, tell Him your plan. It's not really funny but God's plan can be quite different than ours, even laughable. As I look back over my life, what I envisioned never happened. God put all the twists and turns of my life on the right path despite my faulty thinking. I kept running around in circles and was shipwrecked doing it my way. When I finally let go and let God, I could experience smooth sailing for the first time. He has the master plan and the part we play in the big picture is all in the harmony God intended.

If we are discontented it may be a good thing. It may be a signal you are not on the right path, be it in your work or your relationships. Through the help from your Higher Power, you can find a solution to your discomfort and make a God inspired change. When you are doing the right thing you automatically feel better. My job is to keep in close contact with Him in order to be in harmony on all levels of my life. If you are in the wrong job, down deep you know it. If you are in a toxic relationship your gut tells you to get out. I believe your intuition is really your heart trying to tell you the right move to make next.

A wholesome discontent with failure and frustration is incentive for action on your part. Your true calling, since you are one of God's favorite kids, will not be fulfilled until you answer the call.

STEWARDSHIP

We entered this life naked with nothing in our possession and we will leave the same way. When you really boil it down, we never "own" anything. We are stewards of some God given gifts. We have essentials for living for just a short time. It all will go away eventually. "Ownership" is a myth. I really don't own a house or a car. I am a temporary steward of a few material things. Fear is either, fear of losing what you have or fear of not getting what you want. If you really have nothing and trust God to provide your needs there is no reason for fear.

I am not advocating throwing all you have into the trash. It would be prudent to be very good stewards of God given gifts. If you use these things for good, positive purposes you are in service to your family and the community. If you have "stewardship" over 50 acres of land and you grow rice to feed your village, this is a generous use of this piece of land. It really belongs to Mother Earth, not to you personally. We say "my children" and "my wife" when in actuality they are not yours. They are God's kids. When it comes to relationships, no one has "stewardship" over another human being. That's slavery or hostage taking. Sooner or later all of us are going to be detached from all material stuff and relationships, only our spirit will remain.

I have had the experience of losing all my possessions when I was overrun by the enemy. I had my life which was much more important. Stuff is not important. God will provide.

May 22

Look Beyond the Words

The life of recovery has taught me to slow down and look beyond the words. We talk about "one day at a time" constantly. It is not a trite saying but an important concept. My morning prayers, if I read them like rote it would only take 5 minutes. However, it takes me about one hour because I look beyond the words. I stop on different words and phrases every day. I think about how to put the concepts into action as I plan my day. One phrase can keep me inspired all day long. Consider the Lord's Prayer. The first two words, "Our Father" is an entire thesis. "Our" includes everyone. Father explains the relationship clearly.

Much of spiritual literature is just openers for a deeper message with an entire world of thought behind just a few words. Slow and easy is the pace I use when reading. If not, I would fly right by what I need to learn. Also, I have learned to get outside help to interpret words or phrases I don't understand. I rely on Emmet Fox to explain words in the bible. His lifetime of study is available for me to read. It makes better sense than my uneducated analysis. Words change meaning over time and new words pop up all the time. Look beyond the raw words into the real meaning intended.

As time passes and I read the same spiritual messages, I realize I have changed. This opens new horizons beyond the words. I know only a little but a little bit more each day.

SELF-CONDEMNATION

I hear fellow members beating themselves up all the time. We have expectations for ourselves but when they are not met, we get a resentment with the person in the mirror. Of all the resentments we get, at least we can do something about the way we view ourselves. It is just another aberration of self, like self-pity and plain old selfishness. Put self-condemnation to the constructive versus destructive test. It is destructive to run yourself into the ground. Comparing yourself to others is also a form of self-destruction. Your insides will never measure up to the outsides of others. How you measure yourself is the only important test.

If we are doing what we should be doing, it is all we can ask of ourselves. God knows you are giving your best effort. We need to keep a positive attitude about our progress, stumbles and failures. My failures have taught me more than education could. A mistake can always be a lesson, a positive one. If you get impatient with yourself, this will only drag you down. Treat yourself like a wise parent treats his child. Loving firmness without grand expectations will bring positive improvement. We are our worst critics by far. Loving friendly criticism is better than harmful denigration. Be a good friend to yourself.

Mentally beating ourselves up creates a spiral of self-criticism and self-blame. We deserve better. Optimism and encouragement, we do deserve.

SEX PROBLEMS

It was bad enough I had to stop drinking but then the literature said, "we all have sex problems." My reaction was, "How do they know?" None of your business. As I listened to my fellow members, I heard relationship problems meshed together with sex difficulties. Then I came to realize since we all were selfish types. We would have problems because when it came to sex, we were in it for self-gratification. In my spiritual readings, they say hell is unfulfilled desires, hungers and thirsts. We learned booze could not fill the void we felt. Also true with food, gambling and sex. Nothing will patch up a spiritual void except spiritual healing, we finally came to realize.

We drink too much, we eat too much, we need sex too much. We do everything to excess. Even good things, we work too much, we exercise too much, we overdo even the right things. When any of these things becomes an obsession, there is a deep problem. So many of us have to find other help in the area of drugs, eating, gambling and sex addiction. No matter the problem, love is the answer. Prayer is the answer. There is no love involved in selfish sex and the satisfaction is temporary. The craving comes right back. Our minds and bodies become warped in a downward spiral.

Don't worry, pretty soon you will be so old you won't know what I am talking about anyway.

THE JOY OF BEING

Have you ever stopped and contemplated how wonderful it is to just be? For the next ten minutes forget about your aches, pains, problems, relationships, possessions. Just focus on the miracle of being alive at this moment. Forget about time and location just realize the kingdom you reside in. You are the absolute monarch of your own life. Your consciousness confirms you have life. We are sure God wants us to be happy, joyous and free. Just reside in your body. Focus on all the amazing functions in operation to sustain continuation of even more life. A true joy.

If you will look at your gratitude list, you can appreciate the gifts of being. For ten minutes "wants" do not exist because supply and demand are equal. God has provided all the requirements of being. There is no void, no blanks to fill, no emptiness. The baskets are full, the cups are full. Just being is feeling love and nothing else, pure. God is love; and he that dwelleth in love dwelleth in God and God in Him (John 4:16). Just realizing being, recognizes God as the giver of life, a joyful life.

If you put God first in your life, you will not find yourself laboring under anxiety about anything. Total faith. Just being can keep you connected with God. You can feel the joy and love. It is truly staying in the now.

MY ENEMY, MY FRIEND

My biggest enemy was me. I hated myself and really didn't want to be around me. I sought lower companions to be with anybody but myself. I hated to look in the mirror to shave because I saw a pathetic bum. The evidence of my drinking was on display. Black bags under my bloodshot eyes and a puffy face. No matter where I tried to hide, I was with my biggest enemy and I could not shake him. I would pretend I was invisible. I would hold my breath in elevators to not spread the smell of booze. It was horrible being chained to my worst nightmare...me.

Finally, I got "shot down" by my last drunk. I had to raise my hands in surrender. The enemy was now caught in the rat trap. I was still the person I hated the most to start with. Slowly through the steps, my Higher Power, the fellowship and a great sponsor, I began a new relationship. No longer did I scream and swear at myself. I learned to trust myself and felt so much better mentally, spiritually, and physically. I was able to form meaningful relationships, even with myself. After some years I was able to be a friend to myself and enjoy my company. I had many things to learn requiring a positive and happy attitude.

Be good to yourself and be a good friend to you. Buy yourself some flowers. Don't wait on somebody else.

A LOVING GOD

A lot of us, me included, had a concept of fear associated with God. Eternal damnation awaited the sinners and non-compliance with the commandments would be punished in fire. The priests would point fingers and shout fearful messages of guilt and shame every Sunday. I am blessed to hit a bottom hard enough to bring me to the rooms of AA. I learned I could fire my old concepts of a Higher Power and communicate with a Higher Power of my own understanding. I need not accept someone else's God. My elders taught me the difference between religion and spirituality. The best idea was, God wants us to be happy, joyous and free. I now know the truth.

My spiritual teachers confirm what I have learned as a result of being in recovery. God not only loves me but He is our Father, a loving parent. If I ask my Higher Power who has all power, He will assist me with whatever my needs are. Slowly, through what I learned in AA, I was able to say honestly, I have a God centered life. At the beginning, my spiritual life was AA centered which worked well. Today I still have AA as part of my daily life but the center piece of my spiritual life is God centered. Prayer and morning meditation feeds my soul with the strength to handle life on life's terms.

All childhood fears of my past religion went up in smoke. I am on a joyful, love-based journey without fear and guilt. I can feel in my gut I am on the right path.

MAN IS A SPIRITUAL BEING

If you agree human beings are spiritual beings then it is clear a spiritual path is the right one for us. In the bible, an often-quoted passage is (Matthew 6:24) "Ye cannot serve God and mammon." The word *mammon* is the Hebrew word for money. For us it translates not only to wealth but also power, prestige and excesses of all sorts. Emmet Fox explains, "Man is essentially spiritual, the image and likeness of God, and therefore he is made for the spiritual basis, and he cannot really succeed on any other." I have tried the material path already. It did not work for me. From practical experience, I can confirm what Emmet Fox says is true.

There was a time when I had it all. Outward appearances looked fantastic, house on the hill, position of power, wealth but my insides were in total pain. There was a black void in my soul. A vacancy nothing could fill. I tried alcohol but the hole in my soul let even booze leak through me with no effect. My spiritual bankruptcy was deep, dark and complete. I am truly blessed to have experienced and survived spiritual decay. Today I am on the right path, a spiritual path. I have seen both sides. The difference is difficult to describe. You have to live it for yourself.

I am certain the path I have chosen is right because life is wonderful today. It feels right when I try to do the next right thing. God has provided everything I need. No more void, emptiness or anxiety.

CHECKLIST

Pilots have a regular routine of following a checklist. Many a pilot has been embarrassed when he goes to retract the gear on takeoff. Oops, the gear won't come up because he forgot to pull the safety pins. I almost lost a fellow combat pilot over enemy territory. He screamed for help because his engine had failed. He failed to check his oil cap and it came off in flight. His engine seized up as a result. Checklist not done, obviously. My life has always been one of checklists. Today I have a spiritual checklist I perform before takeoff. I don't want to forget important items to insure safe flights and happy landings.

When I wake up, I thank God for one more day of life. Then I start my checklist with prayer. I don't miss this step just like I don't forget to put my feet on the floor before standing. The 11th Step Prayer reads just like my aircraft checklist. It tells me what to do if I encounter hatred, discord, error or doubt. My required action is to bring love, harmony, truth and faith. Check. I have another checklist prayer called Take Time. Take time to read, play, pray, be friendly, laugh, give, work, and think. Check. Another daily prayer has a list of must do items: give every living creature I meet a smile, forget the mistakes of the past and press on to greater achievements of the future. My spiritual checklist gets faithfully done each morning. No exceptions.

I would never try to fly an aircraft without carefully accomplishing a safety checklist. Likewise, I would not launch into my daily activities without reviewing the positive actions I need to do. I have not crashed and burned yet.

To Thine Own Self Be True

I was presented with a 30-day coin. It said, "To Thine Own Self Be True." I had no clue the meaning of the statement. I had been true to just about everybody but myself. The great part of recovery is the concept of starting your life over, only this time with principles. When I did my inventory and examined my motives in early life, I saw a trend of running away. I left home to be a priest but the motive was not a calling. It was a desire to get out of the house. I joined the military, not for flag and country, but to get out of town. I was a misfit from the git go and took on the role of a maverick. It was fun for a while. I got away with a lot of mischief. It all caught up with me because of my drinking.

Thanks to finding the rooms of AA, this do over in life taught me to do what my heart directs. I can reject conventional wisdom and the bidding of others. Freedom to be me, the honest to God me, is high on my gratitude list. Coming to live in Thailand was a big step in following my heart. Today I am picking up a pen and paper to become the writer I wanted to be when I was eight years old. Starting over as a sober person with goals and dreams makes me young at heart and full of enthusiasm.

If you are doing the wrong things with the wrong people, in your heart you know it is not right. It takes courage to stop the insanity and begin anew. The rewards are worth it.

LESSONS OF A FLOWER

Many spiritual readings focus on the lessons from nature. Even though humans are the highest form of life on earth, God has given us clues and lessons we should learn in other forms of life. Some are hints of what not to do. For example, the baby elephant is convinced there is no escape from the small rope around his foot for his entire lifetime. We have the option of gaining freedom from any bonds. We have to change our old ideas. Animals give us lessons but even a simple flower has powerful messages for us. When I want to think of God, I visualize flowers. They are His handiwork for our enjoyment. God's artwork if you will.

A bright orange and yellow flower facing the sunlight is like a reflection of the cycle of life. The flower grew with the help of water, nutrients from the soil and sunlight. Now the flower stands tall on its stem for you to see and take in the beauty of God's creation. It all started from a small seed with roots forming to absorb the energy from the ground. Some water and sunlight bring growth from the small seed to a magnificent flower. Similarly, our faith starts as a mustard seed but it is enough to start the growth process. Then you can stand tall. You are the beautiful person God intended, just like the flower.

Unlike the animals and flowers, we human beings have many choices. We can sustain our growth and reach the highest level God has intended for us. The Sunlight of the Spirit is available to all of us.

June 1

THE ART OF BEING QUIET

I have often written about being a good listener and the noble option of keeping your yap shut. This time I call it "art" because there is a fine line of speaking when you should speak and the times when it would be better to remain silent. I was in my local coffee shop when a tourist came in talking loudly, wearing no shirt, upsetting the management and the other customers. I wisely did not say anything. The manager of the coffee shop gave me the twirling crazy in the head gesture. I thought about the times I did the same thing at parties, making loud conversation and being the center of attention. God was giving me some payback.

I have learned the painful lessons of speaking when I should have been mute. I had many amends to make in this area. When I had a position of responsibility there were times, I told large groups things I later deeply regretted. Some people still quote me from 40 years back. Once you let it rip, it is out there in stone forever. On the flip side, if I can say something to help a suffering soul I should speak. I should speak encouraging words. I should give a positive example of my experience, strength and hope in AA meetings. I should not hog the time from other members. Being labeled a "quiet person" is a good tag. It shows a kind listener.

In my daily prayers, I ask God to guide my speech. God, help me understand I need not comment on every subject. I pray I can open up and shut up at the proper times.

June 2

OPEN MIND OPEN HEART

When I enter a room full of strangers, I look for someone who has a smile on their face. A smile attracts me. Usually, I find a kindred soul for friendly communication. Being an open person makes you truly attractive. Hopefully, open-mindedness is in your tool kit from working your program of recovery. Even deeper is an open heart as part of your character. Open to new ideas, open to others, open to being teachable. I stand with open arms in the sunrise every morning and accept God's love. I try to pass love on to every living creature who crosses my path.

Part of getting into the "open" mode is eliminating self-ishness from your life. If you truly are thinking of others, it will show not only on your face but in all your actions. Some folks naturally are comfortable opening to strangers where others are more reserved and closer to the vest. I changed from introvert to extrovert somewhere in my teens. Maybe even loud, overbearing and obnoxious at times. Hopefully, I have backed off those ugly traits and still am approachable. In AA, I want the newcomer to ask me questions and feel my willingness to help. Every person I have sponsored saw in me an openness. I try to be someone who listens without judgment.

This business of open mind, open heart is key to sponsor-ship in AA. I have been close to the guys who chose me as a sponsor. It is a bond only found in recovery.

June 3

ONE WITH GOD

In our spiritual readings, we come upon passages about being "one with God". The clearest wording I have ever seen comes from Emmet Fox, "First, that God is our peace; next, that not only are we and God one (all spiritual teachings say that) but it is He who has made us one." Fox is explaining Ephesians 2:14 which discusses the wall of partition describing the times communication is broken between God and ourselves. You know how important communication with your Higher Power is to prevent a partition going up, cutting you off from the Sunlight of the Spirit. Once we engage in anger, resentment or any destructive behavior, we are going against God and our true nature.

We are human beings, not able to stay on a straight line of spiritual progress at all times. Once we realize we are on the wrong path we need to stop. We can retrace our steps and clean up any damage we have caused. We can look at the character defects which erected a partition between us and God. Now back on the spiritual path once again we have learned our lessons. Our mistakes can help us build character and make permanent moral changes. Those of us in recovery, have the steps to bring us back in line with God's will for us.

In my past, I was off the path of spirituality for decades. I am forever grateful I survived the excursion into darkness. I was able to bring down the partition between me and my Higher Power.

June 4

I DON'T KNOW

In the old days, it was impossible for me to utter the words, "I don't know." I could hold forth on any topic with great authority. Just ask me. My ego was so inflated. If I was ignorant in a certain area, I would make something up. Current events, world politics and business, I was the expert. Thank God I got leveled in recovery and learned to say, "I don't know." I say it a lot. For the guys I sponsor, I can't tell them how to stay sober. I can only explain how I did it. I stay out the news business and all other normal topics folks like to discuss. I no longer desire to show off my knowledge to elevate myself. When you get older, any expertise you had is now expired.

Learning to say "I don't know," is just one key to honesty, humility, inner growth and new knowledge. If I stuff my ego and ask questions, I just might learn something. If I remain quiet and train myself to be a good listener, I might learn even more. All my former delusions of grandeur have been exposed as BS. Appearing stupid is OK with me if it is the truth. From page 164 of the *Big Book*, "We know only a little." The depth of my ignorance has no bottom. The more, I learn the dumber I get. As I study, I open new areas of ignorance.

When you think about it, saying you don't have the answer is a wonderful freedom. I can seek answers elsewhere. I learn to respect the knowledge and opinions of others.

KEEP MOVING

Folks like us cannot afford boredom for too long because it is dangerous. Lulls in the action breed selfishness. Pretty soon it is all about you and sloth is toxic. Once it seeps into depression it is hard to pull yourself out and get back into the sunlight. Boredom is a dark, lonely place and it can be the circling of the drain. Being alone can be serenity especially in prayer and meditation. But with a negative attitude and isolation from your Higher Power it becomes a problem. A quiet mind is a good thing when I am learning and concentrating on constructive thinking. If I slip into self-pity, self-delusion and fears, then I am in trouble.

Sometimes, no action is the best action, but it can be habit forming until we become spectators on the bench of life. AA stresses getting into service. Action. Thinking of others. I have a regular routine of things I do in addition to the alone quiet stuff. I get to a meeting every day and do all the stuff to make it happen. I get off my butt and get in the gym and do my exercises. If you start your day by one good action, such as making your own bed, you have accomplished something. It will lead into the next action and get you moving. When I feel lazy about doing something, I just start small. Once I get moving then the flow comes along until I finally complete the task.

My energy levels vary greatly. Once I get on a roll, I try to get as much done as possible.

June 6

OWN YOUR THOUGHTS

We are powerless over people, places and things but nobody can control your thoughts. Even if you are in prison unable to be free, unable to make choices, still your kingdom resides in your thoughts. My step-son, Tam did not make it out of Vietnam in 1975 with his mother. The government put Tam in a "re-education" camp for five years. They tried to control his thoughts and forced doctrine to brainwash Tam. They failed miserably. Tam would fall asleep during lectures. At the five year point the authorities allowed "graduates" to go free. Tam was not on the list but when he had a chance, he joined the lineup and walked out the front gate. Now a fugitive, he managed to escape Vietnam by boat.

A long story to the make the point, even a five-year concentration camp cannot steal or control your thoughts. If you allow others to invade your thought-life you are giving up a precious freedom. You might not own anything material in this world but you do own your thoughts. My prayer and meditation connect me with my Higher Power. It insures I am not alone in my thought-life. I do have the power to control and select my thoughts. This freedom is gold. I refuse to let outside influences invade my thoughts.

My thoughts can lead me to God. Good, constructive actions follow from a loving attitude of gratitude. This precious freedom is on my gratitude list.

WHO SHOULD GO ON MY LIST?

Step Eight is just making a list. Simple, right? Many folks have difficulty with this task. What I tell my guys is, put down everyone whose path you have crossed. You owe amends to all of humanity. The idea is to be all inclusive and not exclusive. Get them all, people, governments and law enforcement. It is only a list. We can address the how in Step Nine. There is no statute of limitations for Step Eight. "Oh, that relative has passed away." You're not off the hook because a person is not available. I wrote many letters of amends to persons not alive to hear my plea for forgiveness.

My rule is, if I can remember the event it needs to be addressed. If it bothers me, it must be cleaned up. I said a hurtful thing to a classmate 55 years ago. I got a big laugh to feed my ego. I never saw this guy again my entire life. It still bothers me. He is on my list. His name is Steve and God has put many Steves in my life. I make quiet amends to each Steve as they pop up. I have sponsored four Steves. I add an intensity rating on a scale of one to ten. Amends power of ten went to my ex-wife and mother of my four kids. For years she endured my disease and terrible moves in pursuit of my career. I could never make enough amends. I tried my best until she passed at an early age.

My everyday life is one of indirect amends to all those people I can never reach. I drove a bulldozer through life for 35 years. What a mess.

June 8

FREEDOM, LET ME COUNT THE WAYS

Freedom has so many levels and different aspects I find it difficult to list them all. The freedom you feel from doing amends is way up there. It is like being released from prison after a life sentence was overturned. If you carry your past around without doing something about it, this could be a life sentence. The freedom coming from a cleanup of wreckage is all about forgiveness, restitution and love. It gives your faith a boost upward. My goal is to be weightless. Carrying a bag of regrets and damage was too heavy for me. I dropped the bag of rocks.

If it bothers you and you still think about it, put it on your list no matter how small. Here is one bothering me. Maybe I will feel some freedom if I confess. When I was flying as the commander of a crew of eight airman, I had a staff colonel flying with me. In the air, I was the boss but on the ground the colonel outranked me. He thought my attitude was unprofessional. We made a stop in Saudi Arabia. To taunt the colonel, I drank an imitation beer in the airport snack bar. The bottle resembled a Heineken. The colonel got red in the face and angry, mission accomplished. It took a lot of convincing there was no alcohol involved. I never saw colonel again. It pointed out flaws in my ego and about a dozen more character defects.

My living amends is to be sober and not be flippant. I still have some devil left in me. Old guys need not be boring. The freedom to be silly.

June 9

I Can't, He Can

At the beginning a simple explanation of the first three steps made perfect sense to me. "I can't," for the first step admitting powerlessness. Accepting my life was unmanageable and admission of my alcoholism. "He can," the realization a Higher Power could do what I couldn't. Acceptance my way was insane and only a force outside of myself could restore me to sanity. "I think I will let Him," demonstrating a willingness to let this Higher Power run our lives according to His will. The three small phrases are unconditional surrender and the terms of the surrender. I have passed on this simple summation to the guys I sponsored.

As you know from my writings, Emmet Fox has given me many topics to discuss. The title of one of his meditations, You Can't, But God Can, gave me goose bumps. The reading following this title was exactly along the lines of the first three steps in our recovery program. This is not the first similarity I have found between Emmet Fox's and Bill W.'s writings. Some of the wording is identical. We are blessed neither Bill W. or Emmet Fox advocated a particular religion. AA is meant to be all inclusive but many religions are exclusive in some ways. God is available to all of us, I truly believe.

The more I study spiritual principles, I find the basics are not complicated. The truth is simple and clear. "Let Go Let God," a simple phrase, but it speaks volumes.

June 10

I WAS, I AM

One of the biggest hurdles to my recovery was separating who I was from who I am. In recovery the focus needs to be on who I am today. If I keep talking about who I was, I am repeating history stories. My problem when I first got sober was, I wanted to tell the fellowship who I was. Not a brand new, suffering alcoholic. In my early sobriety I was in a meeting on a Navy base. When it was time to share, I told a story about flying in combat. I wanted them to know I wasn't always a loser. Later one of the Navy guys came up to me and said, "Mike, I really like your story especially the part where you said you were an alcoholic."

The Navy guy gave me a lesson I never forgot. Today, I am an alcoholic. Long ago, I was a pilot. What I am today is the only thing relevant. The members in the fellowship are only interested in how I stay sober today. How I deal with life in real time. Yes, my past may help somebody but I need to focus on lessons learned not pump up my ego. I am blessed some things from what I was are still who I am today. I was a father. I am a father. Hopefully I am a much better father in my sober life. God has given me a chance to improve on what I was over to who I am.

I am an alcoholic. I am an active member of AA. I am happy joyous and free. What I was and who I am are entirely different, thank you God.

June 11

OLD HOUSE OR A NEW ONE?

Raw sobriety is so sad to witness. Members who are sober but it is obvious their recovery went no further. They put down the drink and stopped right there. They are not happy joyous and free. They have not changed one bit with the exception they are sober. Raw sobriety. They have no sponsor, nor do they sponsor anyone, not in service, never talk about the steps and do everybody else's inventory but their own. They are content with the status quo as in living in their old house. The old place is in poor repair. It is like living in squalor spiritually. I might note being sober beats the alternative, but it is a bare beginning.

The *Big Book* talks about a long period of reconstruction ahead. Let me suggest you can build a new house and abandon the old wreck. We have a design for living called the 12 Steps. At our disposal is the Great Architect, our Higher Power. All we have to do is ask and be willing to change. We have the tools in our spiritual kit to do the job right. We have everything we need to build a new life from ground zero. A new house many times better and stronger than your old house. The new one has lots of room for expansion. The old one should be condemned but some folks still live, in disarray.

Are you still an angry, unhappy person even though you have been sober for some time? May I suggest moving out of your old house and begin a reconstruction project. You have everything you need to begin today.

June 12

GROWING INTO WHAT'S RIGHT

We may need to grow into the right path of action or thought. When I decided to move to Thailand I had to grow into the culture, customs and food. Many of the Thai ways seemed strange to me but over time the wisdom of their way became clear to me. Giving is a basic Thai tradition. I have come to believe this trait is better than taking. An even simpler example, Thai food. I don't see too many overweight Thai people so I grew into the Thai diet. Some dishes looked unfamiliar but they were great. Most restaurants have a foreign selection in the front of the menu but in the back is the Thai food menu. I find the right stuff for me there.

Apply this thought to your recovery program. When I was given the AA schedule of meetings I balked. The last thing I wanted to do is go to a meeting. Meetings were a way of life in the military. I had an aversion to the time wasting I endured for years. Lucky for me, my first meeting changed my mind instantly. All my preconceptions were wrong. Likewise, I had to grow into some of the steps which seemed unnecessary at first glance. I could see my fellow members doing all the steps. I knew they were on the right path. All I had to do was follow their example.

My life was always in turmoil and I was accustomed to chaos. In fact, I was hooked on adrenaline. I had to grow into peace and tranquility, a much better path.

June 13

THE SKY IS FALLING

"The world is going to hell in a hand basket." "We are destroying our planet." "The sky is falling." We hear this stuff and doomsday reports all the time. In my youth, I remember WW II was raging and today the world is in much better shape. I believe the world is getting better, just look at the miracle advances in medical areas as evidence. We, as a whole, are living better and longer. Fear not, The Captain is on the bridge. There is no such thing as the perfect storm to sweep us all away. The seas do get rough. If we stay connected to the Most Powerful, calm waters will return.

"Be not afraid of life. Believe that life is worth living and your belief will help create the fact." Quote from William James. Recently a fellow member decided life was not worth living and he died in despair. It is all in the attitude. We can let fear run our attitude into darkness then eventually into death. Fretting over stuff out of your control is robbing you of precious time you could be doing positive things. The world is not going to the dogs. The human race is not doomed. In fact, humans have found new ways to improve life and survive in a changing environment.

As faith increases those fear mongers selling doom and gloom get silenced in your life. You are free to enjoy the Sunlight of The Spirit.

WHO'S RESPONSIBLE FOR THIS MESS?

When I review my past life, I can see clearly my idea of responsibility was severely warped. When the teacher returned to a messy classroom and asked the question, "Who's responsible for this mess?" Nobody would confess and the code was to not rat out the guilty parties. In the military the sergeant would scream at the privates, "Who's responsible for this?" Knowing there was no reward for honesty or taking responsibility, all of us remained mute. As a result, we all got punished. As I matured, I took on responsibility not mine to take. As a representative of my country in uniform, I took on the sins of my superiors. I was guilty for loss of life in Vietnam. Yet my personal life was a mess where I should have shown responsibility.

I was taking responsibility over stuff which I had no control. I was failing to be responsible in areas clearly my responsibility. Then, in our disease, we dump all responsibility and become victims. Everything at my bottom was somebody else's doing. Instead of carrying the weight of the world, I avoided stepping up to the plate for anything. One extreme to another and both were wrong. This program taught me to be responsible for my own actions. My recovery and my happiness are all in my basket. When there is a mass shooting, I'm not marching for better gun control. Not my business. I have plenty of AA responsibilities to keep me busy.

In the morning when we divide up the tasks, I give the impossible stuff, like climate control and wars to my Higher Power. I do the possible things for which I am responsible.

June 15

TRUE PARTNERSHIP

In the drinking days the word partnership was not in my vocabulary. It was all about severing myself in divorce, getting fired and cutting off my friendships. Finally, severing myself from my family and the human race at large, my isolation was complete. In my early recovery, I read this quote from the *Twelve Steps and Twelve Traditions,* "The primary fact that we fail to recognize is our total inability to form a true partnership with another human being." How did this happen? This statement was so true. In my spiritual readings the root cause hit me between the eyes. Selfishness. My isolation was caused by my total selfish behavior.

In recovery, some partnerships came fast and are still in place since the first day. My first meeting I was told this should be my home group. The first man I met said he would be my temporary sponsor. They told me the only requirement for membership is the desire to stop drinking. There were three partnerships right there even though I was not ready to do my part in these partnerships. Quickly I declared the first group to be my home group, the first man I met became my sponsor and I have been an active member of AA ever since. Over time I was able to grow into doing my part in these relationships. Being in service, giving of myself replaced my old selfish behaviors and allowed me to be a fully vested partner.

As far as a partnership to share my life with, even more time was required. I wasn't ready for a true partnership until I had 10 years of sobriety. It happened when God said I was ready.

June 16

EASIER ROAD OR STRONGER LEGS

Many of us are looking for an easier softer way on the road to recovery. We seek a better job, a more attractive mate to share our life with, a new location called "paradise". My spiritual teacher suggests focusing on being a stronger person rather than finding a smoother road. Instead of looking externally for an upgrade we can improve ourselves as first priority. If we strive for harmony and peace, we can take the actions to make them happen. Much better energy spent than searching for the easy way. We do have control over the improvement of body, mind and spirit. If we make our legs stronger, we can handle any road condition.

When we continue to pray and ask God each day to become a little bit better our prayers will be answered. I can handle situations today which baffled me years ago. But it wasn't me, it was God doing for me. Every day I have choices and I try to ask myself, "Will this help me become better?" When I go to the gym, I look for exercises to make me stronger. When I order food, I can choose a salad over French fries. Fruit over a slice of cheese cake. When I have time to read, I can pick up a spiritual book. There are dozens of choices every day and only some of them make me a better person physically, mentally or spiritually. I have found the stronger I am the easier life becomes as the result of improving myself.

I am so grateful that I can make healthy choices today. I need stronger legs because I have many miles to go before I sleep.

June 17

ARE YOU A GRAVE ROBBER?

My spiritual teacher asked this question. I must admit I am guilty as charged. What he is referring to is digging up old resentments and bringing them back to life. We do this by talking about them and rehearsing a list of wrongs about events long past and buried. I shared in a meeting about a family member and listed her sins. I'm keeping my resentments green instead of leaving them buried in the past. What I need to do is have a loving statement if someone brings up this family member. Something like, "I hope she returns to family events and enjoys the love the rest of the family has to give." OK, I will save this thought.

At a family event recently, someone brought up a family member knowing everyone has strong feelings on the subject. I successfully laughed and changed the topic. Resurrecting stories from the crypt is not helpful or useful in any way. No one has seen this person in many years. Another area needs to stay in the ground also. Past operations and sickness need to stay buried and not be rehearsed over and over. Us old folks tend to talk about our hospital experiences and show our scars to our friends. Be happy, joyous and free this moment instead of showing reruns of our operations in colorful descriptions.

My spiritual teacher says, "Don't disturb the dead. Leave them alone." I want to be looking for improvements. I need to quit digging up graves of all sorts.

June 18

NO FAITH, NO LOVE

Fear blocks us from everything but most of all love is not possible when driven by fear. Our faith has to be restored in order to address our fears and give love a chance. When you break fear or lack of faith down, you can see it is inward looking. For example, if you in the survival mode afraid of losing your life, all you think of is yourself. Understandable, but most of our fears are based on selfishness. It is all about you, what you want and think you need. No love is possible. Thinking of others has no priority for people full of fear and lacking faith.

As fear is inward, love is outward in nature. Thinking of others, being in service, giving of yourself are all forms of love. Love can be constructive. It is a positive force to bring harmony and peace where necessary. If faith is missing in your life there is no defense against the many fears out there to invade your thoughts. You against the world is a tough road to travel. Trust me on this one, I tried it and it almost killed me. I can recall times of all fight and no love. A dark and lonely place with no way out.

The solution is simple, acceptance of the presence of God. He is available to all of us. God is Love and my faith gets stronger every time I contact Him. As a result, my life is jam packed with love and little fear.

June 19

LIMITLESS PROMISES

I was asked to comment on a spiritual reading titled "The Last Promise." The reading was about a promise "God is doing for us what we could not do for ourselves," from page 84 of the *Big Book*. Some 80 pages later on page 164 it states, "See to it that your relationship with Him is right, and great events will come to pass for you and countless others." Is this not a promise? My AA Grandma, Alice taught me there are over 50 promises in the *Big Book*. My job is to find them all. The *Big Book* is our personal bible. For an alcoholic, it is clear, written in understandable language. I see things this year I didn't see the year before. I have found about 40 promises and not found 50 plus yet because I have more chambers to open and to see limitless promises.

Many meetings in AA we read The Promises from pages 83-84 which lists 12 promises in one paragraph. Some tend to think this is all there is. Not so. A promise gives us hope if we stay on the path of recovery great things will result and we can confirm this in our own experiences. Therefore, the *Big Book* has scattered many promises to keep the hope alive. On page 164 there are ten promises alone. Can you find them all? It is my belief there is no "last" promise. But there is a continuation of hope and facts which will come true for us.

I constantly review my *Big Book* and declare myself a student rather than an expert. I do realize I know only a little. There is one more promise.

June 20

ASSOCIATING MYSELF

I am forming an association with whatever I allow to enter my thought-life. Most inputs I can control by what I read, what I listen to and who I associate with. I associate myself with AA people, the literature and attend the meetings of the fellowship. I am giving mental assent for all the ideas AA has to offer into my thought-life. This works well for my recovery. I opened the door to let AA into my life. It was my choice and I exercised my freedom to associate with this program. Obviously, this has been a positive, worthwhile association but it can go the other way also.

I do not associate myself with a political party. Those who do pick a particular party have a choice to be constructive or destructive with their views. As a bystander to the drama, I hear a lot of rhetoric about destroying the opposing party rather than the positive actions to be taken by their chosen party. If I join a hate group, I make the principles of the group part of my life and endorse the group. I did belong to what appeared to be group with positive goals and service oriented. However, every meeting was full of anger, finger pointing and rancor. I voted with my feet and left the group quietly.

Emmet Fox says, "Give your assent only to truth." I believe what I assent to becomes part of my life. I carefully choose my associations.

June 21

SPECIAL PEOPLE WITH WINGS

Angels are people who touch your life in a special way. They might not appear often thus you should cherish the times an angel crosses your path. Angels either inspire you or change your life for the better. I have many angels in my life and I think of them with great love and gratitude. One angel worked in the education office where I was taking night classes. He casually mentioned a new program where students could be sent to college and become officers. A few weeks later, I was in the program at Syracuse University. I became an officer with a college degree. I never thanked this angel. He changed my life dramatically for the better.

One of my aunt's sent a handwritten letter to me in the mail. It arrived the day I had a car accident while drunk. She pleaded with me to get into recovery. She was the one angel on the planet who could get my attention. It triggered the process for me to quit fighting and seek help for my alcoholism. The biggest turning point of my entire life. I had angels give me a pass when I should have flunked a physical exam or busted flying rules which would have terminated my career. Angels are forgiving and bend the rules.

I live with an angel who insisted on a trip to the hospital I was refusing. The doctors were surprised I survived a severed bowel. This same angel saved my life again when she spotted a yellow look I didn't see. I polish her wings every day with love and gratitude.

June 22

WHAT HAPPENED TO YOU?

I love getting this question. Friends I haven't seen in a number of years are shocked when they see me. Maybe the loss of 50 pounds helps. Most of them notice I don't have a drink in my hand. Every photo of me from the old days I have at least one hand with a drink. Also, the photo will show me with my mouth open holding forth on something I thought was important. I have never seen a photo of me listening. My friends ask, "What happened to you?" I stopped drinking is the simple answer but it goes deeper. "Did you get religion?" No, in fact I gave up all my old religious ideas for spiritual principles.

The biggest difference they see is a personality change. I no longer need to be the center of attention. I am 90% quieter than anyone remembers. Some even mention a new smile and improved happy attitude. The tough question is, "How did you do it?" The real answer, the truth, I didn't do it. My Higher Power did it. On my own I was going nowhere. The second part which is easier to explain is, "I had to ask for help and I got it." I could talk for hours on what happened. When it is appropriate, I break my anonymity and talk about my life in AA.

Now my friends cannot say, "Mike is still a wild and crazy guy. Drunk as usual." My honesty about what happened to me has led to some sponsorship opportunities. I am grateful to answer the question, "What happened to you?"

FEAR OF DEATH

My spiritual teacher tells me of all the fears one could have, the fear of dying is a waste. If you have faith in God while you are alive what's to fear? The same God will be on the other side when you pass and will still love you the same. There was a time when I did fear death because I had children to raise and fences to mend. Down deep in my soul I knew I was not ready to transition to the other side with clean hands and straight eyes. In combat, I saw death all around me and I accepted death as a probability. I feared being in a Hanoi prison getting tortured for years. Also detoxing in captivity would be hell. Death would be the softer way out.

My son Mike faced death with a smile and a great positive attitude. He did not have one ounce of fear through the six years he endured ALS and he set the example for our family. The bond of love and prayer can bolster faith in God to remove fear. In recovery, I prepare a departure plan every morning in my step work. One more day is OK with me. If I keep my inventory clean and detach myself from material stuff, I am free to travel to the next phase.

Emmet Fox explains you are the same person when you pass on to the next plane as you are now. God is the same, you are the same thus nothing is different. The condition of your spirit is all important on departure.

June 24

LOVE CONNECTION

Two guys are sitting on the subway in NYC. One says, "I'm from Queens." The other says, "I'm from the Bronx." The first one says, "I'm a Yankee fan." The second says, "I'm a Met's fan." Finally, the first guy says, "I'm a Republican." The second guy says, "I'm a Democrat." These two found three differences in the first New York minute and nothing in common. They gave each other the finger and went their separate ways. OK New Yorkers don't be offended. My example would not be likely because on the NY subway nobody talks to one another anyway. My point is we often seek differences rather than common ground.

We folks in recovery are blessed because no matter where we travel, we can find a love connection by attending an AA meeting. Once we enter a recovery room we are with birds of a feather. Everybody there is an alcoholic. We have the same purpose and the same principles. Even if the meeting is in a different language we feel at home. It has been my experience AA people are the most helpful folks on the planet. We all have a love centered life and you can feel the connection immediately.

The same two guys are on the subway but this time one says to the other, "I noticed your tattoo. Is that your daughter?" The second guy says, "Yes from a photo on her seventh birthday." The first guy says, "Wow, I have a seven-year-old daughter too." They chatted, exchanged phone numbers and hugged each other. Hey, it is my story. You knew it had to end with love.

June 25

TRUST

There was a time when I could not trust myself to stay sober. I would break promises to myself to not drive drunk. When I hit my bottom, there was no trust with anybody or anything. Faith and trust went together from rock bottom zero. I did trust my fellow members in AA and they told me to find a Higher Power of my understanding. Slowly I trusted myself to stay sober for one more day. In service for AA, we are trusted servants and I could appreciate the honor of being in service. Then with self-trust and faith in a Higher Power I could address trusting others.

In my spiritual journey I learned we are all God's children. We are brothers and sisters. Trusting my family is basic to normal living today. I have strong trust in my fellow man and on rare occasions the trust is broken. I keep a positive attitude on trust. I found it to be a two-way street. Others trust me to be there when they need assistance. Being trusted is part of love in my mind. My openness makes me vulnerable. A small risk to take versus a suspicious, negative attitude on trust.

If honesty and openness are part of my fabric, others will sense my character and treat me accordingly. I will always be a trusted friend. People expect me to keep doing the next right thing. I will not let them down.

June 26

THE MAGIC PILL

The chemicals we put into our bodies can cause great harm. Take something simple like a packaged dry soup where you just add hot water. The one I am looking at has 25 different ingredients, most of which I have never heard of before. If you want to diet, check out what is in the processed food you have been eating. You will lose your appetite for sure. Then the magic pill roller coaster. Taking an upper. Oops too high, take a downer. Some of the drugs we ingest are solid rocket fuel alcohol. Two of my close friends went from the pill to vodka in a flash. It is my belief there is no magic pill.

I hear folks say their doctor prescribed a particular drug as a cop out. Whatever you put into your body is your responsibility, no matter what. You are the boss of your medical care. I have to be careful because not all medicine works as advertised in my body. I examine any chemical drug or remedy with a sharp eye and test a small quantity first. Mixing different chemicals or drugs can be a real problem. Two drugs may be great by themselves but poison when put together. The less chemicals I ingest the better. I think of God and pray when I get a headache.

There is no chemical solution to a spiritual problem. Just like alcohol, there is no magic drug to make my life better. My Higher Power is the Great Healer.

June 27

THE RIPPLE EFFECT

We have a Thai niece up in the village who is causing a ripple effect throughout the entire family and the neighbors. Her anger and actions have the whole village of 200 people on edge. One person can cause bad ripples or good ones. Once we take action, it may have ripples we did not consider. When I was in college my son watched my study habits and copied my routine. He, in turn, graduated college with three degrees at the top of his class. I had no idea he was watching me. A good ripple effect but I wonder how many of my bad habits also rippled the wrong direction.

The point is, our actions go beyond the initial act. Good deeds are never lost. AA is a prime example of a ripple effect now into its 85th year. From two men to millions all over the globe without a promotion campaign or high finance. One alcoholic working with another is our basic action. Since it is love based it works for us members in recovery. It is not connected to any company, politics or cause. It remains pure in the simplicity and has a spiritual basis instead of a material motive. I feel the ripples in every meeting I attend.

In the year 2100, I pray a recovering alcoholic can trace his sponsor back to me sponsoring one of the guys I work with today. He won't know me but God will. I never know who is watching me as I travel the Road of Happy Destiny.

June 28

MEASURE OF SUCCESS

Of all my old ideas, the measurement of success was totally in left field. I could not be more wrong about what success really was. I wanted to make the cover of *Time* magazine. If Robin Olds could do it so could I. He was a fellow combat pilot with a lot of bravado and accomplishments. I considered myself to be in the same league and I even had a big wide mustache just like my hero. I thought the next higher rank would be success. To make a million dollars was my idea of financial success. A movie star wife would help the picture I was trying to paint. Not one spiritual goal was on my list of what success should be.

My alcoholism made all my ideas of success go up in smoke. I realized all my success goals were about my ego, power, prestige and wealth. How sick can one person be? Absolutely none of my ideas of success survived after doing the 12 Steps. Today I measure success in 24-hour segments. Nothing grandiose on my list of successful accomplishments. Staying sober one more day is success. Working with another alcoholic is success. Being in service to my group is success. I could go on but you get the idea.

Success is not something I need to concentrate on. I turn my life over to my Higher Power and think of others with the idea of being helpful. Success, like happiness, is a byproduct of doing the next right thing.

June 29

RETIRED REBEL

Being a non-conformist was part of my persona. I went to great lengths to be different. I wanted to be labeled a rebel, a maverick. My teenage heroes were all anti-establishment. I was booted from the seminary for an "extreme case of worldliness". A perfect tag line for me. I tried to live the life of a rebel. The military is all about conformity. Well because of the circumstances of the Vietnam war I was able to go off the ranch and be a creative, non-conformist. They have special assignments for crazy guys like me. I broke every rule. Never followed the crowd. Somehow, I got away with my non-military behavior. Becoming a drunk just added fuel to the mixture.

When the military returned to normal, I wasn't normal. The curtain came down on my rebel act. Nothing worked anymore, booze quit working. My behavior wasn't working either. Lucky for me AA didn't come on strong with conformity or else I would have walked out. I needed some direction because I was lost. My sponsor had a plan for me and I followed his direction. I went to a meeting every day, assumed a service position and did the steps. Conformity was working miracles in my life. I dropped the attitude of going against the flow.

Today, I'm a retired rebel conforming to all sorts of things. My days of tilting windmills are over. I try to comply with God's will for me and drop the fighting attitude.

June 30

COMPLETE ENLIGHTENMENT

The Dalai Lama is one of my spiritual teachers. One thing he says I totally accept, "The task of man is to help others; that's my firm teaching, that's my message. That is my own belief." Simply stated a single task. Our AA program is in line with the Dalai Lama in singleness of purpose. I truly believe my only job for this life is to help others. Then reading on, the Dalai Lama has this to say, "As long as you are not completely enlightened there will always be an inner obstruction to knowledge that will make your task of helping others incomplete." Am I completely enlightened? I am moving in the direction of more knowledge. To claim to be completely enlightened, no way.

Since I will never be completely enlightened, I will never reach fulfillment of my main purpose in life. I have come to the conclusion if I keep seeking, learning and trying to help others, I am on the right path. If I do the best I can then I know my Higher Power will understand. I probably miss little opportunities to help others every day. I could have tried to make a sad person happier. I just passed by and said nothing. The task at hand is open ended. I can always do better.

What can I ever do completely? I can stay completely sober one more day. I do not expect complete enlightenment but I get closer every day.

A WALK IN THE WOODS

My spiritual teacher tells me if I am in pain to think of God. If I am struggling with any kind of problem, I should not focus on the problem but focus on God as I understand Him. I do just what was suggested by wiser souls. The process works wonders. Everybody has a different image they pull up as they think of God. My method is to think of nature as an expression of His artistry. I believe there are messages in nature for us to learn. Deep in the woods, where no one lives, nature is growing vegetation and fruit. Birds are tending to their young. Caterpillars are turning into butterflies. All beautiful forms of life.

A walk in the woods alone puts me closer to God. I soak in the artwork God provided for viewing. There are so many places on this earth far from the reach of humans. All of it is God's universe. I am in awe of the creatures in nature surviving and sharing the wilderness with thousands of other species. When I take my walk, I can see how insignificant I am in the bigger scheme of things. Just another form of God's creation. My problems seem so trivial when I absorb the power of nature.

In my flying days I saw a good portion of this planet from high altitude. There are vast areas uninhabited to be alone with God. I recommend a walk in the woods to experience God's gift for us to enjoy.

July 2

SURPRISES

I had a boss who would often say, "No surprises. I hate surprises." He had a bad attitude in my opinion. Being a bit evil, I decided to change his negative view and give him a big surprise. I hired a singing telegram for his birthday and planned a surprise birthday party. He kept his birthday a secret but my spies had access to his records. The surprise would be even better. I picked up the attractive singing telegram and brought her to the party. Sure enough, my boss hated his surprise. All the office loved it. My boss glared at me and shook his finger at me. I pleaded innocence. The cake and ice cream in his honor did nothing to quell his wrath.

Life would be a bore without surprises. I expect them often. One of my daily prayers says, "expect only the best". I look for good surprises every day and I seem to find them. Once or twice a week I see old friends in my home group meeting from years back. Renewing friendships is a loving surprise. I gave my five-year-old Thai nephew a 500-piece jigsaw puzzle. He was surprised and happy. The biggest surprise was nobody in the family had seen a puzzle before. I gave my angel a surprise party for the first time in her life and she loved it.

Surprises amount to expecting changes out of the blue for the better. I try to surprise the people I love in a good way. It is a creative expression of how much I care for them.

July 3

BECOME A CHILD

"Except ye become as little children, ye cannot enter the kingdom of heaven." Quote from *Twenty-Four Hours A Day*. Right now, I am enjoying my five-year-old Thai nephew in his innocence. A child seems to have strong faith which fades with maturity. The Thai family of eight all sat down for dinner at our local restaurant. My nephew sat with me. When we ordered Thai dishes, he said he would rather have what I am having, Italian carbonara. Independent and trying to learn new things. What a joy to observe youth blossoming. His first trip to a beach made me feel young. He jumped for joy splashing water and doing flips. Unbridled energy.

My nephew's visit charged my batteries. He inspired me to become a child again without being childish. Life is simple to the child and I need to seek more simplicity in my own life. My nephew loves to eat shrimp. At the restaurant his mom gave him some small shrimp from her dish. Not acceptable. He said, "The ocean is right here, I want the big shrimp from the fisherman." Smart as a whip and wants the best. He looks me in the eye and wants to learn from me. He did give a thumbs up on the carbonara by the way.

I pray I can be a child in faith with a sense of fun and play to offset the burden of every day chores. Little children love so openly and freely. My nephew gives me genuine love hugs. I am grateful for the lessons he has taught me.

July 4

HAPPINESS AND HEALTH

My spiritual teacher wrote a piece about happiness and health I found inspiring. He suggests good health will naturally follow from happiness. They work in harmony so aches, pains and soreness are not part of a happy person's life. An unhappy person is much more likely to be sick and physical ailments will be part of his list of complaints. My teacher's theory is to focus on being happy and your world will be a joyful one. Happiness, I learned a long time ago, should not be pursued as an end to itself. Happiness comes as a by-product of doing the right things. Our program puts us in perfect position to be happy through the process of the 12 Steps.

My teacher explains, "God has a plan for every man, and He has one for you. Your real problem—the only problem you have—is to find your true calling in life. Everything else will fall into place." Ask yourself, have I found my true calling? I asked myself this question after completing the 12 Steps and the answer was a resounding, no, not even close. I was pretty far down the road to seek a true calling. But with willingness to change, I found it. I know I am on the right path now. I can feel it on several different levels just like my teacher describes. I am doing the right things for the right people. I am happy with myself.

If you are on the wrong path, down deep you know it. If you have doubts why not ask your Higher Power for help? When everything is in harmony, happiness and heath will follow.

July 5

DISCONTENT

Discontent may not be a bad thing. The road of life gets bumpy for all of us. We are not content 100% of the time. When a period of discontent arises the advice of my spiritual teacher is to deal with it as soon as possible and be done with the problem. Our goal is to dump discontent in minutes, not days or months. God wants us to be happy, joyous and free. I want what God wants too. First question, do I have any control over the situation? If the answer is no, we can pray for acceptance and change our attitude toward the discontentment.

Discontent can cause us to take action and maybe change our priorities. If we are off the path God intended for us, we should feel discontent. We need to do whatever is possible to unblock the road. If you have a resentment brewing, my teacher tells me I need to go see my brother and resolve the matter. Now, not next week. My natural tendency is to avoid my discontent with this person and forget the fact he is my brother. I need to resolve the matter with love and not in anger to make the discontent worse. My spiritual teacher says I might as well deal with it now. If I don't resolve the problem, it will carry over to my next life.

Emmet Fox says, "A wholesome discontent with dullness, failure, and frustration is your incentive for overcoming such things. Whoever you are, your true place is calling, and, because you are really a spark of the Divine, you will never be content until you answer."

July 6

SWEET FREEDOM

On my gratitude list I have freedom down twice. Freedom from the bondage of alcohol. Freedom to have choices. Actually, I could list 20 more freedoms to my list. We have so many freedoms we take them for granted. They are part of our everyday life. The freedom to tap into my Higher Power whenever I want, for as long as I want, is worth more than gold. Nobody is forcing me into a religion, some cultures do. I can choose my significant other, some places the spouse is designated without your permission. Everything I eat I can choose, hopefully what is best for my health. Freedom of information is part of our lives today. Nothing is withheld from our thirst for the facts.

We have many freedoms we don't exercise. We are free to travel endlessly but we choose one location to live. Our freedoms are gifts we should be grateful for and protect them from loss or harm. Our freedom from prison or bondage should not be at someone else's expense. Freedom is to be shared with everyone. Modern technology has expanded our freedoms beyond the imagination of a generation ago. We are free to communicate, real time, with voice and images anywhere in the world. An amazing boost to love connections with family and friends.

All of these freedoms we enjoy have responsibility attached. It is easy to expand our freedoms past their intended use. I pray I may remain grateful for the gifts of freedom and put them to the proper use as God directs.

July 7

SPEED

"Everybody should be free to go very slow." Quote from Robert Frost. As a reformed speed freak, I learned some things are better by slowing down. I kept falling down in my daily exercise walks until I admitted my mind is younger than my body. Now people on crutches pass by me on the sidewalk. In fact, I get pushed aside on occasion when I go too slow for folks in a hurry. Everybody has their own speed for what they do. They should be free to go the speed which works best for them.

In the business of recovery, I do encourage the guys I work with to keep moving forward and not take it too easy. Years ago, I was sponsoring three guys at the same time. They all had less than a year of sobriety. I picked them all up and we went to meetings together like a big happy family. After a while it became clear to me, they were at different speeds in recovery. I needed to work with them individually, rather than as a group. Their needs and problems were quite different. I was slow to get into recovery. I got here later than most. It's not relevant anymore because I made it. Some call recovery slowbriety.

The old story of the race between the hare and the tortoise we all know well. Not only did the tortoise win the race but the tortoise lived four times longer than the hare. This is a message.

July 8

EMPATHY AND ACTION

Most of us consider ourselves to be compassionate and sympathetic. These are great emotions to have but what do we do to show empathy and care? Unless these fine emotions lead to action it is hot air. There is a Thai saying, I will loosely translate, "sweet mouth, sour results". In other words, flowery, flattering speech is covering up the true sour actions. Good intentions are wonderful as long as there is follow through. "I intended to make a meeting today. I intended to be in service but something came up." I hear this often when I run into fellow members who have been missing from the fellowship.

Feelings of sympathy and compassion are important to possess. There is a responsibility attached to these feelings. My heart is calling to reach out to those in need. My only job on this earth is to help others. I need a daily action plan to fulfill the task. If I am consumed with selfish pursuits, I don't have time to reach out. I walk right by opportunities to be helpful because I have blinders on. I have been self-absorbed to the point of not responding to old friends and hurt their feelings.

From the Dalai Lama, "True compassion is not just an emotional response but a firm commitment founded on reason. You develop a feeling of responsibility for others; the wish to help them actively overcome their problems." Yes, I am responsible.

July 9

MOVING DAY

In professional golf tournaments they have a term "moving day". The tournaments last four days but after the first two days the field of competitors is cut in half. The ones who do not make the cut go home with no prize money thus "moving day". We have something like golf when we do our 7th Step. We move from our own stuff into helping others. We become useful, maybe for the first time ever. Lucky, we don't have a cut line in AA where we send people home. I make the cut every time I help someone.

"The Seventh Step is where we make the change in our attitude which permits us, with humility as our guide, to move out from ourselves toward others and toward God." Quote from *Twelve Steps and Twelve Traditions,* page 76. We need those first seven steps to prepare us for moving into the realm of helping others. I remember my first moving day. I was the literature person for my home group. I came to the meeting place at 6 a.m. one hour early to set the books out. I opened the room, turned on the lights, cleaned up all the leftover whiskey glasses and beer bottles. I arranged all the chairs for the meeting. I changed a bar into a nice meeting place. It felt good to be useful to my group. I did the meeting set up for years after.

When I move from my selfish pursuits into being of service to others, it is a "moving day" for me. The further I am away from myself the better I feel. The closer to God I become.

July 10

BE A PARENT

"Hey, Mike I don't have any kids." Yes, you do. Your inner child you keep beating up. My spiritual teacher stresses treating yourself as a loving parent would. Handle yourself as a wise parent handles a child, patiently, but with gentle firmness. It is harmful to be too hard on yourself. If you are doing your best then God understands. Being impatient with yourself is counterproductive and foolish. As long as you are not lazy or complacent you are doing alright. Early in sobriety, when I was frustrated with myself many members told me, "You are right where you are supposed to be."

I really like the idea of treating myself as a wise parent in other matters also. I desire improvement and it hurts when I have a behavior relapse. Some character defects I thought were long gone pop up unexpectedly and I curse myself. Why did I argue over nothing important? Mike the adult, can tell Mike the child, "You forgot to pause before you opened your mouth Mike. It will be OK, no big deal. Forgive yourself and press on." Much better than the old days with real parents, a beating and being sent to bed without supper.

We are our worst critics. Expecting the best is part of my morning prayers. I also accept my human failings and give myself a break. If I trip and fall, I dust myself off and keep going.

July 11

RECIPROCAL JUDGMENT

"Judge not, that ye be not judged. For with what judgment ye judge, ye shall be judged." (Matthew 7:1-2) We all understand the law of gravity. Reciprocal judgment is a cosmic law just as true as gravity. We can try to ignore this law or argue our special case. My spiritual teacher tells me whatever judgment I apply to others the same judgment will be applied to me. It may be delayed but a day of reckoning will come. Judgment is part of human activity. We make judgments about people and situations. Quite often we do our judging on partial information. We usually don't have all the facts.

A quiet mental judgment in the privacy of your own mind is one thing. When this judgment leads to action we could be in danger of harm. Recently a man lost his life while being arrested. A fact, but add this to the fact, a black man lost his life while being arrested by a white police officer. Now we get a whole new set of judgments and plenty of action. Get the media involved to fan the flames of hate and racial unrest. The judgments of thousands of people replaced the judgment of law and order. The result was burning buildings, breaking glass and defacing property. One wrong multiplying into countless more wrongs.

Misplaced judgment or incorrect judgment can be extremely destructive as we witnessed. Where is love and peace in the scenario I have described? The cosmic law was broken.

July 12

GIVE ME RECOVERY OR GIVE ME DEATH

Back in 1775 an American patriot, Patrick Henry, gave a famous speech where he delivered the line, "Give me liberty or give me death." We in the fellowship can paraphrase this famous line; give me recovery or give me death. For us, to drink is to die. Most of us hit a turning point. Go to the bottle and die or turn your life over to the care of a Higher Power and recover. Maybe on the doorstep of death. One more drink could have punched my ticket to hell. Through the grace of God and a sliver of willingness, I crawled into recovery with the Grim Reaper on my shoulder. I could have missed the beautiful life I enjoy today. It was close.

In the end, we have two choices. Keep on destroying ourselves and damaging our loved ones or seek help and surrender. The alcohol route took away all my ability to choose. Demoralization was a polite way of describing how I felt. I was clueless about what the life of recovery would be like. I was painted into a corner with no way out. I simply said out loud, "God help me." And He did with my claw marks in the floor all the way to my first AA meeting.

I pray I may accept the challenges in recovery and be grateful for escaping death. May I use this extra time I have been granted to help others.

July 13

HUMILITY LESSONS FROM THE DALAI LAMA

In our recovery literature we read, without some degree of humility, no alcoholic can stay sober. Step Seven is focused on humility. I take several actions every day to insure I stay humble. I look to one spiritual teacher to learn more about humility, the Dalai Lama. I read from his book, titled *The Path to Tranquility*. His quote contained in the Forward of the book is the same message I have for you in my writing. His quote, "I humbly pray that readers may find some inspiration in these words to develop that warmhearted peace of mind that is the key to enduring happiness." The next section, Editor's Note, contains *Eight Verses for Training the Mind*. I will highlight a couple of the verses on humility I found inspiring.

"When in the company of others, I shall always consider myself the lowest of all. And from the depth of my heart hold them dear and supreme." Quote from the Dalai Lama. I was taught from the beginning when I enter a gathering of people, such as an AA meeting, to consider myself the most unenlightened person in the room. In fact, I am not any "est" at all. Not the smartest, richest, or best in any measure. Back to the concept of "just another bozo on the bus".

The next verse from the Dalai Lama gave me food for meditation. "When others out of envy, treat me with abuse, insult me or the like. I shall accept defeat, and offer the victory to others." This goes against my instincts. A lesson in humility I pray I can apply.

July 14

JOIN THE INSANITY OR NOT

There is an old Irish joke I heard years ago. An Irishman looking for a drink entered a pub and walked into a big fight in progress. The Irishmen took off his coat and inquired, "Is this a family fight or can anyone join in?" We may on occasion be faced with a decision. To join a fight or not join the fray. Family problems are so difficult to deal with when emotions are out of control and our loved ones are involved. My policy has always been to not take up one side over another no matter what. When my mother and father were going through their divorce, both of them demanded my active support. I refused to pick one parent over another. They both cut me off, which was a good thing at the time.

Remaining calm when pots and pans are flying through the air is a challenge. Duck. But if you throw one pot you become part of the problem rather than the solution. My gut feeling in family disputes is to play the role of peacemaker or referee. Even good intentions can go sour. Not adding anything may be the best route and remain silent. Displaying calm can set a peaceful example. Pray some of the combatants follow your lead. I know if my anger gets involved, all is lost. I become useless and pour gas on the fire. Love is the answer.

Arguments and turmoil always have some elements of fear. If you can do something to dissipate one those fears in play it may cause the entire argument to unravel. My parents accepted my love again once the storm passed.

A NEW YOU

When I first got sober the folks in recovery before me stressed, I should find a Higher Power, of my understanding. I did just what they did and found a brand-new concept of God. It works well why not adopt a whole new me of my understanding? I saw where all my old ideas would result to nil. I stay in the now and don't waste time agonizing over the past. What's left? A new day, a new beginning, new ideas, all resulting in a new me. I want to be happy with me. To accomplish the level I desire, some changes need to take place. Improvements in body, mind and spirit are all possible with the help of my Higher Power.

I must always remember how powerless I am. God has all power and all I need to do is connect with the power source through prayer. Ask and you shall receive. Look in the mirror. Do you like what you see? If not set some body goals. Diet and exercise can always be improved. Is your spiritual bank account low? Get in more service, go to more meetings, read more literature, work with other alcoholics. Is your mind idle, without meaningful inputs? Read some spiritual books. Turn off junk TV and put your phone down. The new you deserves the best. You can start remodeling right now.

You can carve out a designer you to be the beautiful person God intended. If your life and heart is full of love you will radiate. Every day brings a new, improved you.

July 16

SHARING MATH

"Trouble is part of life, and if you don't share it, you don't give the person who loves you a chance to love you enough." Quote from Dinah Shore. Every year when I read this quote it inspires me. It makes me grateful for the opportunity to share often. We humans are social animals and crave connecting with other people. When we share our joys with our loved ones the happiness is doubled. Likewise, when our sorrow and pain is shared the agony is halved. The math in sharing is always in our favor. I was taught to keep my troubles to myself.

My old tendency was to stew in my own juice. No more, with a group who knows me well, I can share my ups and downs with ease. I let the sharing math work for me. If I am troubled my loved ones wrap their love around me and comfort me. I feel better. They feel good for the opportunity to help me and love me even more. During my hospital visits and operations, I witnessed love above and beyond by my wife. She took charge when my decision making was impaired. She ran a tight ship and I felt safe, protected and loved.

Stuffing my feelings does not work for me. The magic of the fellowship is part of my daily life. I don't take it for granted. I share my life openly and enjoy the multiplier effect of love.

July 17

REPETITION

"Repetition is reality, and it is the seriousness of life." Quote from Soren Kierkegaard. I have found spiritual fitness is enhanced by repetition. I say the same prayers every day with a pause and focus on a few phrases as I go. I know my prayers work. I need to keep on repeating the process every day. If I get off my routine it is hard to get back in the groove. Using exercise as an example, I travel five miles on a treadmill as my routine. If I stop, nothing changes for a few days. But all of a sudden, my weight jumps up three pounds. It then takes weeks to get my weight back down. I keep up my repetition because the penalty is too great for a lapse in my regular exercise. Being overweight puts me in danger.

In my spiritual fitness, my peace and serenity are at stake. If I drop my daily connection with my Higher Power the sky doesn't cave in the next day. However, slowly the different spiritual actions of my regular routine get replaced by negative, counterproductive actions. The decay is insidious but eventually a relapse will happen. Maybe not a sobriety relapse but a spiritual, emotional or mental relapse. Pray, go to a meeting, talk to another alcoholic, or help someone. One or more of those will work for me.

I try to improve by adding, not subtracting, to the repetitions of my day. I am grateful for the balance in my life. It took years of hard work to find the right combination.

July 18

WHERE IS GOD?

One of my spiritual books has this line, "We can believe that God is in His heaven." People look up or point up when they refer to God. To my belief, God is not located somewhere else. He is here all around us. God is all things and all life. God is in every one of us. We are His children and He has made us part of His kingdom with all the privileges of the human family. God is there for all of us, all the time. We can connect with God anytime. All we do is ask. "Ask, and it shall be given to you; seek, and ye shall find; knock, and it shall be opened to you." (Matthew 7: 7-8)

We experience a spiritual awakening as a result of doing the Steps. This is a start toward nirvana the Buddhist teaching describes. The Buddha is "awake" rather than a God or human. Nirvana or heaven is not located somewhere else. Heaven is right here all around us but we are not spiritually mature enough to see it. We don't know our true location in our Father's house. We are not yet "awake". My spiritual teacher stresses we are One with God. When we harm another, we are harming ourselves. When we help others, we are helping ourselves. Golden Rule.

There is no need to travel the earth looking for God. He is here. He is us. Our loving Father wants us to join Him at His table right where we are.

HUMILITY AND GRATITUDE

I talk about a gratitude list all the time. Still, some of you don't have a list or can't find it. The guys I work with can whip it out in a heartbeat. You can't possibly think of all the things on your list all the time. If you have the list in your hand and review the list, as I do, the result is humility. So many of the gifts you have today were nonexistent while you were practicing your disease. All of the freedoms we enjoy are through the grace of God. I see myself as a child of God, spiritually immature. I have a humble start of a new life.

None of the items on my gratitude list are derived from my skill and cunning. They are the result of doing the 12 Steps. I needed help for each step. Accepting I can't do this program alone, is key to my humility. The review of my egotistical past reminds me how pathetic my behavior was in the days of self-will run riot. Ego and gratitude don't mix. Humility and gratitude are like cream and sugar in your coffee. If you make your gratitude list part of your morning prayer and meditation, you don't have to worry about humility. Humility follows from all your spiritual actions.

My only job is to help others. I must do this with the spirit of humility and weakness. If I speak from a moral high ground all is lost. One bozo helping another bozo works wonders.

July 20

VICTIMS

I have been a victim a few times. I got sold a piece of land which turned out to be federal land. Another time I lost promotions because one of my peers stabbed me in the back. Both of these incidents and some others were all part of God's plan for me. Everything came out for the best in the end. We are in the business of helping others. Coming to the assistance of victims is a golden opportunity to put our program into action. I had some rewarding chances to help victims over the years. I see victims of poverty and hunger almost daily. I could not possibly just ignore these victims God put in my path.

There are real victims who need real help. Some play games with the system and look for a victim's payday. Being a victim can be an attitude and mind set. Some blame outside entities when the solution can come from within. Then there are those people who are self-styled martyrs. There is no plus side to martyrdom. Some alcoholics view their alcoholism as a disability. I am a beneficiary rather than a victim. My disease put me on a spiritual path and gave me a new wonderful life.

I pray I may be able to help victims when I can. I try to prevent abuse when I see it. My gratitude list proves to me I am not a victim. The blessings on my list can be useful for helping those less fortunate than me.

July 21

LEARNING TO TRUST

My spiritual teacher specializes in simplicity. Here is a quote, "A universally applicable test for truth. It is a simple question. Does the truth work in our lives?" He explains further, the test is so simple most clever people pass it over. I don't consider myself clever but I missed the point until I dug deeper. Before I surrendered and entered recovery my only truth was, I needed another drink. Nothing else was true. The 12 Steps made me face the truth about myself. Today I know myself, not the fake personality I put out to others. In my search for a Higher Power, I learned God is Life, God is Truth, God is Love. He has all power. I can connect with God through prayer and tap into His power and grace.

In the work of my recovery, I started from zero on truth. All my old ideas of what was true had to be reexamined. I found whole areas of truth I missed until I began my journey on a spiritual path. Combined with a true picture of who I really was and a new understanding of my Higher Power I began to collect many truths. I have just a good beginning. The same spiritual teacher says, "Truth heals the body, purifies the soul, reforms the sinner, solves difficulties, pacifies strife."

All those things my teacher lists have happened to me. To answer my spiritual teacher's question. Does the truth work in my life? I can truthfully say, yes.

July 22

LOVE OVERBOARD

Years ago, a member of my group gave me the nickname of Love Bug. I liked the tag and my day starts with love and ends with love. God is Love. God loves me and all my brothers and sisters. God wants me to be happy, joyous and free. I share my love as much as I can. I have crossed the line in the past. Not only did I love you but I tried to make you follow my definition of love. I expected you love me to my specifications. Love overboard. Real love means accepting you as you are, not as I would have you be.

Right after I finished college, I decided my wife should have a degree also. I decided we should be a power couple to enhance my climb to bigger things. I took my wife through registration and picked her classes. I told her she would love college just like I did. When I came home the first afternoon of her classes, she was sitting on the couch with her feet up. She never went to one class. She gave me her special glare. She just wanted to be a mother not a college graduate. Big resentments both ways. All because I was designing someone else's life in the name of love.

I had the good sense not to try to mold my children. I let them pick their path without my input. They did just great without Pop selecting their education. With my wife, what a horrible mistake I made. She forgave me over time.

July 23

DREAM THE IMPOSSIBLE

When we were kids, we could really dream great stuff. In class, I could be crossing the Rocky Mountains until my teacher slapped my desk and woke me up to reality. I read a lot which fueled my day dreams. Over time all my dreams went up in smoke. The drinking years cut off a lot of things. Dreaming was one of them. I never thought about dreaming as a recovery topic. A few years ago, there was a workshop at our AA convention titled "Dream the Impossible Dream". I thought this was a mistake. Then the lights went on. We stopped dreaming in our disease. Now we are able to resume our forgotten dreams.

"Imagination is more important than knowledge." Quote from Albert Einstein. Knowledge is limited whereas imagination has no boundaries. All progress in technology had to be imagined first before it became a reality. Einstein goes on to say knowledge can get you from A to B but imagination embraces the whole world. I like what Steve Jobs had to say, "The ones who are crazy enough to think they can change the world are the ones who do." In the fellowship, with love and acceptance, our spirits can fly again. Our dreams can be reborn. There is nothing too crazy I can't share with my fellows in a meeting.

In 1994 I had a dream of long-term sobriety, good health and restored family relationships. It seemed impossible. The dream came true by the grace of God. My dream machine is back in working order.

July 24

YOUR EXPERIENCE

"Experience is a hard teacher. She gives the test first and the lessons afterwards." Quote from *A New Day,* page 203. I hope and pray I have learned from my experiences both positive and negative. I have the opportunity to share my experiences in the hopes my lessons will help somebody else. One of the benefits of belonging to this fellowship is the sharing of each other's experience. If I listen closely, your experience can teach me lessons I need not experience myself. A high percentage of alcoholics are also drug addicts. Over the years I have heard many stories about drug addiction. The stories of detoxing and prison will keep me from ever being tempted to pick up.

Your experience can tell me what to do or what not to do when I am faced with the same situation. More experienced members explained to me about entering into a relationship before I was ready and had some sobriety under my belt. I was advised by wise members I would change much in recovery. They said as I grow in sobriety my former relationships might not work. I have changed dramatically. Both these examples were right on in practice. I have learned to trust others. I have an open-mind to hear the lessons they have for me.

In the thousands of meetings, I attended, the fellowship passed on so many gems to enrich my experience level. It's like I lived a thousand years.

July 25

TURNING POINT IN THE STEPS

Many members argue over the order of the Steps. Do we need to do all twelve in a certain order? I don't want to enter into a debate. I can see the thought of our founders and the wisdom of how the Steps are structured. In the beginning of recovery, it is all about you. Your powerlessness, your Higher Power, your inventory and your character defects. Before we set sail on final goal of helping others, we need to do some much-needed work on ourselves. We are not ready just yet at Step Seven. Then, the turning point, God does the work. He chooses which character defects need to be removed before moving on.

Now the entire focus changes from you, since it has been all about you up until Step Seven. From Step Eight to Twelve, now it is all about others. You can't help someone do the steps you have not done yourself. I needed to change and the Steps did the job. It took years for the process to chip away at the old me and mold a new person. I'm not finished by any means. I was able to sustain a relationship after ten years of work. I was able to admit I had taken the wrong path for 40 years and accept defeat and start anew.

This design for living we have I didn't fully appreciate until I put it into action for a few years. Now I see the beauty of the work our founders put into the design.

YOUR BUSINESS, MY BUSINESS

When I was growing up, I had such low esteem I didn't have a humility problem or an oversized ego. Slowly I had some accomplishments instilling some self-esteem. Then when I became a pilot, an ego was born. I was a lowly pilot for a short time but then I got the title "controller". I was working on becoming an alcoholic at the same point. A horrible combination in hindsight. The "controller" title led to a series of titles: director, leader, chief, commander. My business was to make my subordinates follow orders to accomplish the mission. In other words, my business was your business also. Now we have a drunk egotistical control freak.

The responsibility of managing a 64 aircraft operation was no problem for me. Everybody followed my direction. But I couldn't handle my family or personal relationships. I was taking care of everybody's business but my own. When I took an honest look at myself in recovery, it was clear my priorities were upside down. It was like I could solve anyone's problems but I couldn't tie my own shoes. When I read the part in the *Big Book* about the "director" the hair on my neck stood up. There I was in black and white, perfectly described.

The concept of minding my own business had to be learned. It is much easier than trying to force others to do what I want. My goal today is to do the next right thing and mind my own business.

July 27

SEEING GOD

"We practice the presence of God by seeing Him everywhere, in all things and in all people." Quote from Emmet Fox. When I try to think of God, I start with nature. I can see God's handiwork in all the plants, flowers and trees. The array of colors, the varieties of fruits for us to enjoy is spectacular when you think about what is all around us. The animals we share this planet with all have lessons for us to learn. It is amazing how they survive and have a place in our world. Dogs are extra special. They are attached to us humans and happily share their lives by our side. A dog knows how to communicate with us in a loving manner.

I can hear God in rain and thunder. I can feel God in the pounding surf and high winds. I can see God in my surroundings. My sticking point is seeing God in others. It is easy to see God in those with a high level of spirituality, such as the time I met the Dalai Lama. My goal is to see God in everyone and I admit this is difficult. To love my enemies and people who have caused great harm to my loved ones is a goal yet not reached. When I meet someone, I proceed with caution instead of unconditional love immediately. I know God is in all of us thus I need to see better.

I do believe God's presence is in everything and everyone. I keep seeking to increase my love, reduce my fears and sharpen my vision.

July 28

THE AGING PROCESS

The latest item on my gratitude list is old age. Into my eighth decade I consider making it this far a blessing. I would not be here if I didn't find my way into recovery and get sober back in 1994. The outside part of me shows the wear and tear of all eighty years. What hair isn't white is gone, my wrinkles have wrinkles, and my height shrunk several inches. The inside part of me is new. New ideas, new horizons, meeting new people regularly. A happy new day every day is what is happening on the inside. I am as young as I ever was. My insides and my outsides are going in opposite directions.

My mission is to slow the aging process down as much as possible. My body is withering away, as it should. No surprise there. The inside of me is more vibrant than ever before. Through the Grace of God, my life has been saved many times over. I am eternally grateful for another day. I have miles to go, manuscripts to write, people to help, books to read, family projects to complete and living amends to perform. Each day I am busy with doing the right stuff for my body, mind and spirit. I believe a strong mind and spirit can slow the body aging process down.

Time is my friend, not my enemy. If I keep learning and remain teachable, I will stay forever young. I am born again with every sunrise. My future is only 24 hours at a time. Who could ask for anything more?

July 29

NATURAL COMPASSION

"Since we have a natural compassion in us, and that compassion has to manifest itself, it might be good to awaken it." Quote from *Dalai Lama Path to Tranquility,* page 279. If loving kindness is your religion, as it is with the Dalai Lama, compassion is a way of life. My book of daily wisdom written by the Dalai Lama has eighteen references to compassion. The Dalai Lama has faith we all are compassionate by nature. It doesn't always result in action. Our primary purpose of helping other alcoholics who still suffer is all about compassion. We all have been in a dark place before we had an awakening of some sort. Empathy for suffering souls should lead us to compassion.

In the quote there is the word "awaken". It comes up in key places in Buddhism and in our program with "spiritual awakening". We all have great qualities as part of our nature. Some are sleeping and not part of what we do. When I try to help another alcoholic, he may act negatively to my efforts and even get nasty. True compassion is pressing on and not losing my good feelings when the going gets rough. I need to stay loving in my attitude no matter what. I learned as a life guard a drowning man will fight you. You still need to save his life.

When I see a falling down drunk my compassion is awakened. I see myself in the drunk I once was and could become again. I need to help others when I get the opportunity.

July 30

THE PATH OF KINDNESS

Before I entered the world of recovery I was on the path of selfishness. I could not even be self-supporting and take care of myself. Thinking of others was not happening. Finally, when I surrendered and began recovery, they told me I needed to give it away to keep it. I did the Steps, got into service and began to help others. After life got better, my health returned and I was again, self-supporting. I was able to travel to Vietnam, Laos and Thailand on an amends trip and enjoyed the experience. Soon I was spending half my time in Thailand and became part of the recovery community in Bangkok.

In my morning meditation, in Hawaii, I had the inspiration my heart and soul felt more at home in Thailand than in the USA. The people of Thailand smile, always have a soft word and are naturally kind. It is a culture of service and giving. I felt the harmony of where I was in recovery, doing service and helping others. I followed my heart and moved to Thailand. I have been happy, joyous and free since I made the decision. Here I try to do anonymous acts of kindness every day to join this culture I love so much. My smile is my passport here.

There are many ways to show loving kindness without money. Giving is an attitude and a path of life. Sharing and giving of myself is my new normal. My recovery life and my community life are now the same.

July 31

ISOLATION

Isolation for human beings is just not good. For us alcoholics it could be disaster. Of all the stories I have heard about re-lapse most start with "I quit going to meetings." In one word, isolation. The loss of contact with the fellowship. Then losing the program altogether is the next step. The 2020 worldwide virus has given us a special challenge to maintain our spiritual condition by adjusting to our new environment. Isolation can lead to thinking of only ourselves, our problems and cutting off communication with others. It takes some extra work and creativity to stay on the path we have established in our recovery.

Most us could not attend an in-person meeting for a time. I was on the street every morning for years. I was on the way to a before meeting, a one-hour meeting and an after-meeting discussion. Being isolated in my room was no fun but the zoom meetings filled the void. I agree, zoom is not as good as face-to-face meetings, albeit with a mask on. I found time to reach out to friends in and out of the program through electronic means to stay connected. Words of encouragement helped some, the contact helped me. The virus situation brings powerlessness to all of us. If we fight it, get frustrated and lose our serenity, we are in the danger zone. Prayer, attitude adjustment, new priorities are all things still in our power.

I miss the hugs from my friends but I still love them and find ways to keep the love connection alive. I follow the isolation rules. This virus is tough on old people like me. My computer and phone aren't isolated.

August 1

IS THE DOOR LOCKED?

There is an ancient legend from the Middle Ages with a great message. A local citizen was arrested by the king's lawyer and sent to a dungeon for a life sentence. A huge, fearsome jailer with a key around his neck threw the citizen into a cell and closed the door with a loud clank. Once a day, the door would open for bread and water and quickly slam shut again. After 20 years in the same cell the citizen decided to confront the jailer who would surely kill him and end it all. The citizen went to wait by the door. To his surprise there was no lock on the door and it was open. He walked past two guards, who paid no attention to him. He walked home, joined his family and lived happily thereafter.

The moral is to examine what we accept. The citizen accepted he could not leave his cell but he never tried the door. I know my room was my cell at my bottom. I assumed and accepted I would die a drunk. I couldn't leave my little cell. In my mind there was no way out. In all of our lives, obstacles are placed in our path. My alcoholism was a life sentence in a dungeon of my own making. Thank God I got help, the door opened. I found a way to walk away, join my family and live happy, joyous and free.

Maybe there are some doors in your life you assume are locked. Seek God's help. He may have a window open somewhere. You can bypass the door.

August 2

THE SPIRITUAL LIFE

"The spiritual life is not a theory. We have to live it." Quote from *Alcoholics Anonymous,* page 83. I used to think of a person leading a spiritual life as a man wearing a robe. I now know a spiritual life is open to everybody. To be such a person does not require a religious affiliation. When I entered the doors of AA, I had no idea it would lead to a spiritual life. I just wanted to get the heat off and stop the pain. On day one if someone had said I was now entering a spiritual life I would have run to the exit. Connecting the dots between putting the drink down and being able to honestly say I am leading a spiritual life took a stretch of some years.

The 12 Steps are effective, not only to stay sober, but to change your entire life. You realize the best way to change is finding a Higher Power and getting some help. Then prayer starts small and short like the Serenity Prayer and grows to many more prayers. The literature opens up new ideas about what is truth. I don't know what step I took that crossed the line from an observer of the theory to actively living a spiritual life. Today my day begins and ends in prayer. Everything I do has a spiritual center.

Now I cannot visualize my life any other way. I have found the God I was seeking and know my life is on the correct path. I can feel it in my heart and soul.

August 3

GIVE YOURSELF A COMPLIMENT

We always hear put yourself on your amends list. Forgive yourself and be good to yourself. In a reading from *Body, Mind and Spirit* there is an article on complimenting yourself. It took years before I was able to accept a compliment from anybody. It doesn't happen often but today I can graciously accept a compliment. But give myself a compliment? Something new to consider. I have undergone ego reduction in depth and patting myself on the back is not me. You have heard me talk about buying yourself some flowers instead of waiting for someone else to do it. Apply the same thought to a compliment. It may be many moons before I get my next compliment.

It is my belief you need to actually do something to deserve a compliment. The reading suggests to look at what has happened in the recovery process. I have learned a lot about gratitude, tolerance, forgiveness, faith, love, and prayer. I am in service, sponsor guys, belong to a wonderful fellowship and maintain great relationships with friends and family. Considering I was at death's door at the beginning, I can see amazing changes have happened to me. I did the footwork but had a lot of help along the way. I can sum up a compliment to myself by saying, "You have come a long way, baby."

True enough, it was bumpy at times but look at me now. I can honestly say the gifts on my gratitude list are nothing short of a miracle.

THE ART OF LISTENING

Listening is a special challenge. Not because I don't like to listen but my ability to hear is poor. Between noisy aircraft and old age my hearing aids aren't strong enough. When listening to another person I really have to concentrate and listen with my entire body. I need lips to read and body language to help me. I focus on the person I am listening to in order to get the message. Some voices are out of my range. I hear the voice loud enough but the words are garbled. When I am doing recovery work nothing beats one-on-one communication. Sincerity and attentiveness are key elements to go with the words.

When I say, my whole body I mean I quit attending to myself and my needs. My focus is on listening only. It is all about the other person 100%. I don't play with my phone ever. It is in my pocket and off with no vibrate. I don't sip coffee and look around the room. I maintain eye contact to make sure I am totally connected. The biggest gift I can give is myself, my time and my attention to show I care. More important is what my mind is doing. I try not to think of my own stuff and put myself in the other person's shoes. If I disagree with what the person has to say I keep my argument in storage.

I call it an art because listening skills can always be improved. In the past the voice in my head was always louder than the person speaking. My disability has sharpened my skills.

August 5

THE ART OF TEACHING

I had a few opportunities to be a teacher over the years. I truly love teaching. I'm not saying I'm an expert but the process has been one of my life's enjoyable experiences. Hopefully, knowledge is passed on from teacher to student as a meaningful product. I have spent 20 years of my life sitting in a classroom as a student. I had great teachers and ones I thought were horrible. To be honest I have learned a lot from teachers who I did not like personally. I had plenty of role models before I took the podium myself. The art part of teaching is to connect mentally with your students in a trusting, loving relationship. I think it is helpful to be part entertainer to hold the interest of the student. The process should be fun.

One Air Force position I cherished was teaching pilot instructors the Principles of Instruction. Every class had 16 fellow pilots for the two-week course. I taught eye contact, use of notes and techniques of running a class. I had to practice what I was preaching. It takes two for a meaningful relationship and teaching will highlight this truth. If the teacher or the student has a bad attitude, no learning will take place. Willingness, an open mind by both parties is key to learning. To be a good teacher you have to learn first. My spiritual teachers are my role models.

I also taught college courses for two universities at night. The nights I taught I couldn't go to sleep. I was full of enthusiasm. If I could do my working life over, I would be a teacher.

EMOTIONAL EXPRESSION

One big disadvantage of military life, besides getting shot at, is emotions are not authorized. No time for feelings, just lock and load with your mouth shut. My military bosses never once asked, "How are you feeling today?" Makes me laugh to even imagine it. Stuffing my feelings and emotions were a big part in my drinking. Then booze warped my feelings and it was not the true me. A life of recovery has wonderful, daily opportunities for expression of emotions. I trust my fellowship to listen to how I am feeling and give me honest, loving feedback. What a joy, what freedom. Getting your feelings back is an awakening to yourself.

The next part is difficult. I need to learn how to deal with these feelings muzzled for decades. The good news is now you can do it. The bad news is maybe uncovering some demons you were not aware of. Maybe it is time to get some outside help just like when you first got sober. I spent ten sessions with a relationship counselor. She had some shocking things to say about relationships. I had no clue. It was no wonder I could not sustain a meaningful relationship. The obvious got right past me.

I really had no idea who I was, what I wanted and where I was headed until years into my recovery. The false image or ego had to be crushed into sand. Excuse me, I'm getting emotional.

August 7

LINKAGE

When I was drinking my life was fear driven which made sleeping difficult. I would start with one fear and try to forget about it. Another fear would replace the first one and continue a daisy chain of horror robbing me of peace of mind. No rest for the wicked. There is a flip side, now my life is love based, replacing all those fears. One friend said he has a gratitude list in his head and heart which is good enough. My point has always been you cannot think of all those items at one time. A physical piece of paper can let you see all your gifts at one glance. As I hold my list, I see amazing linkage. One item connects to another to make a chain of gratitude.

The first item on my list is my sobriety. It is directly linked to the grace of God, which led to peace, which is kin to serenity. Today I have choices, which reminds me of my many freedoms such as mobility. Love connects with everything on my list. Specifically, I have love of my children, my parents, my family, my friends, my fellowship and more. My commitment connects to responsibility which connects to honesty and open-mindedness. Everything on my list is linked to other items on the list forming the mosaic of my life, all gratitude based. If I could chart a vector analysis of all the linkage it would cover an entire wall.

You saw this coming, right? Take your list and enjoy the process of linking everything on your list into one chain of happiness.

SENSE OF PURPOSE

Most of my adult life somebody else dictated my sense of purpose. Life happened to me instead of me charting the course ahead. I was adrift in a dingy with no rudder. Now, thanks to the program, I do have a clear sense of purpose. I start my day asking my Higher Power for assistance in my daily life. I need to determine which way God is going so I can go the same way. My singleness of purpose is spiritually centered to stay sober and help others. I have a set of tried-and-true principles to guide me. My prayers outline a number of meaningful goals.

My life, before recovery was minus principle with a selfish center. Helping others is the whole point of living a sober life. A drunk has no time for others. My daily goals are outward in nature. The attitude of giving instead of taking is on my compass for the daily voyage. When the day is finished, I hope I have become a little bit better person. Some good deeds have been accomplished. If I encounter obstacles on my path, I have experience on how to handle the pot holes. I know how to get help when I am baffled. With a strong sense of purpose, I don't stray too far off the path.

I have a firm commitment to my singleness of purpose. No longer do I wake up to dread and fears. Hope, love and gratitude wake me up to face another wonderful day.

August 9

LETTING GO

When I was a practicing drunk, I made a trip from Honolulu to San Antonio. I drank in the airport and the seven hours on the airplane. I joined a reunion of my buddies toasted. I found an open spot on the floor and took a nap. My friends decided to have a memorial complete with candles and a lily on my chest. I was holding a whiskey glass and the gang thought it wouldn't look good in the picture. Try as they might, I had a vice grip on the glass. I would not let go of my glass, even passed out.

Letting go of my alcohol was a tough chore. The next thing was to let go of all my old ideas. Everything about me was old but I finally learned to let go. Then I had to let go of my house and my car in a divorce. My relationship sponsor taught me how to let go of a relationship with love. Lawyers are not necessary in a peaceful, loving parting of the ways. I am really getting into this letting go deal. I let go of my resentments. I let go of my past. After completing the 12 Steps I was on a spiritual path. I started letting go of material stuff in favor of spiritual progress. Letting go is a wonderful feeling of freedom.

A huge part of my recovery was learning to let go and let God. Letting go is a part of accepting powerlessness. If I can let go of the glass in my story, I can let go of anything.

August 10

STANDING STILL

Wouldn't it be great to stop time when you are enjoying yourself? Imagine a gourmet dinner so delicious you want to savor the flavors forever. You can't stop or your food will get cold. In a few minutes the meal is over and you forget the pleasure. Same problem with sobriety. You can't stop time and just stand still. Either you are moving away from your last drink or you are moving toward the next drink. You are moving, like it or not. Like a good cowboy, you need to lean forward in the saddle to progress down the trail. Life is constant movement.

Early in sobriety I tried to stand still. Life was just about perfect. I was healthy again, felt great, and had no problems. I was enjoying the fellowship and going to meetings regularly. Don't rock the boat. Don't fix it if it isn't broke, was my theme song. My spiritual bank account was on empty. I quit working the steps. I was standing still. When a problem popped up, I had a drink in my hand. I couldn't believe it would happen to me. As long as everything was going my way, I was fine. I had no defense over the first drink when I encountered difficulties.

The incident scared the hell out of me. I put the drink down after the first sip. It tasted awful and I felt awful. I called my sponsor and we got busy moving again. I learned an important lesson. I have moved forward since my one slip.

August 11

THE SEARCH FOR POWER

From Step One, we admit our powerlessness over alcohol. The lack of power is our problem our literature tells us. For all of us alcoholics we seem to have misplaced our power source. We were on the wrong power grid. I know I was looking for power in all the wrong places, prestige, money and relationships. There is plenty of power available but our search for power has been totally misdirected. "But there is One who has all power—that One is God. May you find Him now!" From *Alcoholics Anonymous,* page 59. Quote from Emmet Fox, "God in you is greater than any difficulty that you may have to meet."

The search is over. God is not out there somewhere hard to find. He resides in me. I need to find Him right here. My spiritual teachers taught me the best way to connect with my Higher Power is through prayer. I can testify prayer works. Now it is easy to separate where I do have power and where I do not. Makes life much simpler. I have plenty of power to do what I need to do. Stay sober and help others. My tasks and my happiness are all in my power grid. No longer do I waste time pushing power buttons not available to me.

"God can help you in proportion to the degree in which you worship Him. You worship God by recognizing His presence everywhere, in all people and conditions you meet; and by praying regularly." Quote from Emmet Fox *Around the Year,* page 205.

August 12

THE OSCAR GOES TO...

"More than most people, the alcoholic leads a double life. He is very much the actor." From *As Bill Sees It,* page 140. I should have a whole trophy case full of Oscars for my acting performances. I was able to play many roles at one time. None of them were close to the real me. I would put on my costume, a uniform and play the role of boss and leader. I knew my lines pretty well. It was the party line. I didn't have a makeup kit, although I needed one at times. I did have my repair kit, eye drops to get out the red, breath spray and heavy cologne to cover any alcohol odors. OK lights, camera, action.

Instead of an Oscar, I should have been sent to Betty Ford with all the other actors getting busted for addiction. My act was the same role for years. My proficiency at acting was polished by experience. All of a sudden someone yelled, "imposter" and the gig was up. Down came the final curtain on my show. Actually, it was a relief to stop play acting. Thanks to the program and the grace of God I threw my Oscars in the trash. I became authentic. It is much easier to be one person and be real.

Today I can relate to my family, my fellowship and my community with one personality. Now I have one set off principles for every situation and every relationship.

August 13

HUG YOUR RESENTMENT

"If we could read the secret history of our enemies, we should find in each man's life sorrow and suffering enough to disarm all hostility." Quote from Henry Wadsworth Longfellow. I wish I could have seen the above quote during my drinking years. My life before recovery was full of resentments. In recovery, I was taught we are all God's kids, making everyone my brother or sister. We are all related and need to love each other unconditionally. If I can just imagine my enemy as a small innocent child enduring the loss of his parents. Maybe he suffered any number of tragedies of which I have no knowledge. I might be able to hug this person instead of plotting revenge. Resentment always implies some judgment. We never have enough information to pass judgment.

When judging others, we are using our particular set of standards. Our frame of reference may be totally irrelevant. This became clear to me when I did my amends trip back to Vietnam. I judged the Vietnamese to be monsters, evil by nature. I was using American standards in a totally different culture I didn't understand. On my return visit, I learned to love my former enemies. They had more than their share of pain and suffering in a long war. I was just a visitor.

Our program of recovery makes it clear no one is more important than his brother. I wasted years of my life embroiled in resentments.

August 14

GOD IS MY PARTNER

"If you really make God your business partner in every department of your life, you will be amazed at the quick and striking results that you will obtain. Here is a partnership with Infinite Wisdom and Infinite Power awaiting you." Quote from Emmet Fox *Around the Year*, page 224. From only calling on God in emergencies to making Him my partner is a huge leap. The first idea I needed to change was the concept of God as harsh, condemning task master. I now truly believe He is our loving Father wanting the best for all of us. He is available for those who ask and seek.

In God I trust, which is key to the partnership. All my spiritual teachers agree prayer is the best method of communication with God. My daily routine is a conversation with my Partner, my Father who has all the Power. I try to listen to my heart for messages and intuition for the hours ahead. My part in the trust is to do what I know is right and stay in harmony with my Partner. I am confident the Kingdom of God is within me. As a limited human being, I have faults. I make frequent errors but I can connect with my Partner to get back to a spiritual path.

Partnership has many benefits and responsibilities. The weakest member will have the strength of the entire partnership working in his favor. It's a perfect deal for a weak, struggling alcoholic.

August 15

DECISION MAKING

In my past life I made some critical life and death decisions. I'm still here which may lead one to conclude I made the right decisions. I think it is the grace of God keeping me alive, not my decision-making prowess. My decisions were made without consulting my Higher Power. Bad idea. My decisions were made from selfishness. No consideration of others and the effect upon their lives. Most of life's decisions are not of the life-or-death variety. I made career choices for my own benefit. It uprooted my children from schools. I put the pain of moving on my wife's shoulders.

Recovery has taught me to be in contact with my Higher Power at all times. Especially when faced with a difficult decision. The technique I have used for years is sleep on the decision. Say a prayer before going to sleep at night. Let your brain have a rest on the subject. In your morning meditation, more than likely, the solution will come to you loud and clear. In your decision making, be considerate of who else may feel the effect of your action. My decision to move to Thailand came just like I described above.

You have been sober for a while doing all the right things. As a result, your intuition is stronger. You can trust your inner voice. With God as your Partner, you can't go wrong.

PAIN MANAGEMENT

This topic hits home for me. I lost two friends, both with twenty years of sobriety, to problems with pain management. They proved going back out after a long stretch of continuous sobriety is much worse than the first time. Things get really bad, real fast. Both my friends were regular members, in service and going to meetings. It doesn't seem to matter when it comes to pain. I hear, "The doctor prescribed these pain killers for me." Chances are the best doctor in the world may be in the dark when it comes to addiction. If you search hard enough you can find a doctor to prescribe anything you want.

We are not doctors but we are in charge of our sobriety and our health care. One friend was prescribed pain killers by his dentist. He heard the same thing drummed into our heads, "pills are solid fuel alcohol". My friend abused the dosage. He took more than the dentist prescribed. The pills led to vodka. Twenty years of clean and sober time went blowing in the wind. By the time I heard about the problem he was arrested for possession of heroin. He had overdosed twice. He cut off our friendship. He passed away in a flop house.

When I experience pain, I think of God and his presence all around me. I pray. I think of others who have endured much more than myself. I try to get out myself. If I focus on the pain, it gets worse. Pain will pass.

August 17

CRISIS MANAGEMENT

I remember in my early sobriety I read, "Life is not an emergency." I said, "Yes, it is." Life was crisis management for me. It took a while for me to realize most of my emergencies were of my own doing. In the military, crisis is what we lived for. One of my positions was Chief of the CAT, Crisis Action Team. I must confess, I was an adrenaline junkie. I was hooked on crisis to feed my addiction. If you wanted somebody to go behind enemy lines and join a group with 50% mortality rate, I was all in. My blood is rushing thinking about it.

The rocking chair on the porch is where you will find me today. Hard to believe at one time I was the US planner for an all-out air war with the Soviet Union. I couldn't manage my relationships or any phase of my personal life. In recovery, I got out of the crisis business. Today, I tend to my own business. There are no more big deals in my life. This month my biggest problem was my printer ran out of ink. I shrunk my universe from the entire planet down to my tiny office. My task today is happiness management.

The world is in crisis right now. In my opinion, we are not managing it well. I can only do my little part to stay safe and pray for a solution. I got fired from the CAT team and manager of the universe. This is a good thing.

August 18

THE DRUNKENNESS OF ANGER

"The intoxication of anger, like that of a grape, shows us to others, but hides us from ourselves." Quote from Charles Caleb Colton. This quote is perfect for us alcoholics. I grew up an angry young man. It became part of my life and my job. One day I woke up and I was an angry old man. I missed the middle part. Anger drove me because my entire life was fear based. The middle 30 years I was drunk and angry. A formula for disaster, turmoil and confusion. When I am angry everybody around me sees how insane I am. I don't see myself. I am a crazy maniac out of control.

One of the first things I heard in recovery, was anger is a dubious luxury of normal people. I knew I had an anger problem before I got sober. I was a fighter, fighting everybody and everything. My first meeting the speaker said, "You don't have to fight anything or anybody, anymore." The air went out of my lungs. I surrendered right then. I got out of the anger and resentment business as first priority. Anger is a type of drunkenness. I am intoxicated with self, displaying my ego and selfishness for all to observe.

Once an episode of anger is over, my eyes open to broken relationships and broken glass. Anger avoidance is in my daily prayer. It is working well.

August 19

DOING OUR PART

"God gives us the nuts, but He does not crack them." A German proverb. I laugh every time I see this short proverb of real truth. My spiritual teacher stresses helping ourselves in addition to our prayers. If you are praying for employment, it is advisable you write a resume and seek interviews. We need to do our part. My spiritual teacher warns our prayers will be answered but not as we expect. I was taught to do the next right thing and pray. Leave the results up to God. Another caution was not to pray for something impossible.

My case history was similar to the example above. I went to a group specializing in resume writing. I had answered dozens of ads in the newspaper. I even hired an overseas job placement agency. Nothing happened. One morning, after my prayer and meditation, I said out loud, "Dear God, I cannot go another day without a job." The phone rang and it was a former student. He told me they had a job opening with his construction company. Of all the different jobs I could do, construction was not on my list. He set up an interview on the spot. I went with a resume not fitting the job description. I was honest about my lack of qualifications. I got the job anyway.

My prayers were answered in an unexpected field with good pay. The construction job led me to the next job in the area of recovery where I belonged. I did my part and cracked the nut.

August 20

RETREAT

After the years of hard charging, I have learned to retreat when necessary. If I am at a family gathering with a large number of people, I can't handle the intensity of all the conversation for too long. I have learned to find an escape route to retreat into peace, serenity and a quiet zone. This is especially true if drinking is involved. Personalities change, the voices get louder and insanity rules. I'm out of there when I see the mood of the room changing. I use my old age to advantage and excuse myself. I let the younger hard-core drinkers have center stage.

Even at large AA functions, without the alcohol, I need to take a recess away from the ego fest. Pretty soon my stories start expanding into even better stories and off we go. I have learned to take a time out when I feel overwhelmed by too much activity. My inputs are not important. I try to stay out of hostile situations and arguments. I have learned to pick my battles and stay mellow. The Dalai Lama says if an argument is so important to someone angry and upset, he allows the person the victory. It ends the problem. Good plan.

Retreat, in my military days, meant defeat or loss of territory or even an entire country. Today retreat is a personal choice to maintain my serenity. I regroup and take myself out of the fray. I love to miss a good fight.

August 21

THE WASTE OF WORRY

I thank God every day for my change from negative thinking to positive thinking. The sky was always falling in my life. I heard a speaker who said, "I had horrible things in my life and a few of them have actually happened." The actual horrible events in my life were a surprise. I didn't have to waste time worrying about them, they just happened. "That the birds of worry and care fly over your head, this you cannot change, but that they build nests in your hair, this you can prevent." A Chinese Proverb.

Concerns are natural but if worry paralyzes you to the point you get depressed it is a problem. If you have your Higher Power beside you at all times, you have a partner to keep you safe. Worry has two bad sides, living in the future and lack of faith. Worrying will not change the outcome. It can destroy your peace of mind and rob you of sleep. I had an ultra sound test my doctor ordered to check a "suspicious" spot on one of my kidneys. If growth was detected, he warned it may need to come out. I told my doctor, "No problem I have two." He was surprised at my positive attitude. Why worry about it? It is what it is.

The worst scenario of all is worrying about things you have no control over. A total waste of time. The birds of worry would have a tough time trying to build a nest in my hair.

August 22

Tool Kit

My first tool kit was a small canvas bag I used working on B-52's in northern Maine. I was working on the flight line when an ice storm hit. I asked for a truck to pick me up when I finished my job. It was more than a mile away from my shop. Too slippery for any vehicles I was told. I tried to walk but it was too slick to even stand up without falling down. I laid face down on the ice and used two of my screwdrivers like ice picks. I propelled myself up to warp speed and made it back faster than a truck without freezing to death.

Someone told me, "If the only tool you have is a hammer, every problem looks like a nail." Before recovery the only tool in my kit was booze. It was my hammer and every situation got hammered. In recovery, I was given a new spiritual tool kit. My most important tool is prayer. I use it every day. The fellowship has a wrench for every nut in the room. Sometimes I'm the nut, other times, I'm the wrench. Electronics, a computer, the phone, email, are all in the tool kit. Spiritual literature is a tool I use extensively on a daily basis. I'm sure your tool kit has some I haven't mentioned.

I find new tools to add to my collection all the time. No longer do my problems get hammered like a nail. I lost the hammer out of my kit bag a long time ago.

August 23

DAILY TREATMENT

All the month of August I think of my son-in-law, Dan, who passed away five years ago. He had a wound and blood infection that required daily care and treatment my daughter performed for years. His generous loving spirit is part of our family forever. We also have a disease requiring daily treatment even though there is no bloody bandage to change. Even if we do not feel sick or in pain, we must remember we are, indeed sick. If we skip treatment, we soon will feel the effects. It might not be physical, but it could be emotional sickness.

I have a stomach acid problem requiring medicine every day. If I forget my treatment, I will be miserable all day. I don't forget my morning pill. The same with my morning meditation. I treat my illness of body, mind and spirit through prayer, reading my spiritual literature and adjusting my attitude. If I skip this treatment, I would be out of balance for the next 24 hours. My daily connection with my Higher Power is a key element of my treatment. Without God, I am on my own without direction. My disease is progressing. It is not going away. I need to remember this truth.

The problem with the disease of alcoholism it makes us think we are OK. It's a lie, we are not OK. A daily treatment of our disease works wonders. I thoroughly enjoy treatment.

THIS IS BEING RECORDED

One of my favorite teachers, Emmet Fox, has a story titled, *Your Invisible Dictaphone*. He explains everything we say, think and do is recorded in the subconscious mind. A record is in file storage for future use. He suggests if we heard a complete replay of every word we utter in a day, we might be embarrassed. We would be surprised how much negative thinking we do in one day. The brain is an amazing organ to store more information than google.

My subconscious sends my conscious mind information from the past all the time. Sometimes in a dream, which I recall when I wake up. Other times in prayer and meditation, a scene from years past comes forward for review. This is a gift for doing inventory and making amends. As I write stories from 50 years ago, I recall vivid descriptions of events, including conversations. When I was treated for PTSD the doctor put me under hypnosis. I spilled out events from 35 years back in explicit detail. When I came out of the hypnosis I was drenched in sweat. I couldn't stand up without help. I truly believe what Emmet Fox has to say.

I exercise caution and choose my words carefully. I need to apply the same caution all the time because it is being recorded in my subconscious. By the way, this meditation is being recorded.

August 25

INTERNAL DIALOGUE

When I take a walk in my Thai neighborhood, I see a home-less lady sitting in the same spot every day talking to herself. She always has a smile on her face, sometimes laughing, happy with herself. I wish I could be as happy with my own internal dialogue. I chew myself out often and say things to myself like, "You old coot, you forgot your hearing aids again. Go back home dummy." My mind is always churning and yakking away. When I run the tape back, I hear a lot of negative dialogue going on. Sometimes there is a nasty argument happening in my own skull.

When I have a conversation with someone else, I try to be open-minded, loving, and cheerful. Why not apply the same manner to my internal dialogue? Am I not a friend to myself? Some work to do here. In my morning hour of prayer, med-itation and spiritual reading my thought process is channeled in a positive way. The inner dialogue is muted to a great extent. As the day wears on, the good start fades away with events and interface with others. Little bits of negativity be-gin irritating my internal dialogue. I need to give my mind a shower just like my body after exercise.

If I start talking to myself out loud the guys in white coats will come take me away. In the privacy of my own home, I read my gratitude list out loud. Soon I am happy and laughing again. I am not powerless over my internal dialogue.

August 26

THE GREAT MOSAIC

"You are only one part, but an integral part, of God's glorious mosaic." Quote from *A New Day,* page 237. I visualize my existence as one grain of sand on the beach of life. All around me are other grains of sand, some brown, some white and some black but all equal in every way. Up close, sand is not a pretty picture, but draw back to outer space and look down you see a beautiful tropical beach. God is the Master Artist who has the larger picture designed into a wonderful mosaic for us to observe. We are part of the Grand Design.

Yes, we are tiny and insignificant but as Emmet Fox stresses, the Kingdom of God is right here for us, right now. We, the powerless grains of sand, can connect with God who has all power. We cannot achieve great spiritual heights on our own. Through prayer, faith and action, we can. As limited human beings it is impossible for us to see the great mosaic. To know we are included as part of God's plan is a joy. If you can be unselfish enough to look outward and upward, you can broaden your field of vision. I know from flying at high altitude I didn't see garbage, traffic jams, and anger. I just saw the beauty.

When we are having problems and tragedies, it is a good time to remember our tiny perspective. Try to envision the great mosaic. God wants us to be a happy, joyful part of His Universe.

IT'S THE LAW

Laws, rules and regulations always brought out the rebel in me. Breaking rules was my sport, my adrenaline fix. I have a natural aversion to laws and rules. "Know the rules well, so you can break them effectively." Quote from the Dalai Lama. Now there is my kind of guy. In all my years in the military I seldom read a regulation. They were written in obtuse language and invited loop holes. Somebody would let me know when I was violating a regulation. I didn't need to read them myself. But there are all kinds of good laws, and some are more like truth. My prayers will be answered and prayer works. I know this is true. It fits into one of the many spiritual laws.

"I pray that I may submit to the laws of nature and to the laws of God. I pray that I may live in harmony with all the laws of life." Quote from *Twenty-Four Hours A Day* August 26. There are three different kinds of law in the quote. When I read this, I decided maybe I need to drop my law-breaking attitude and learn spiritual law. From the same reading above it continues, "If you are dishonest, impure, selfish, and unloving, you will not be living according to the laws of the spirit and you will suffer the consequences." The 12 Steps have kept me within the law.

"For not the bearers of the law are just before God, but the doers of the law shall be justified." (Romans 2:13) I promise to be a law-abiding citizen from now on.

August 28

HUMAN NATURE

Always in the search for new ideas, I browse my local book store for inspirational material. I found a book on the laws of human nature, so I bought it. Each chapter has a section on the keys to human nature. It highlights our vulnerabilities, weaknesses, emotions out of control, limitations, violent nature and aggression. Then, to my surprise, the book had no spiritual center but suggestions of how to exploit human nature to your advantage. Yikes. You won't find this book on my recommended list. I choose to look at the positive side of human nature.

"An open heart is an open mind." Quote from the Dalai Lama. Open-mindedness along with humility and willingness is the nature we seek. I believe the heart and the mind can connect in a good, spiritual way. "Compassion is not religious business, it is human business, it is not a luxury, it is essential for our own peace and mental stability, it is essential for human survival." Quote from the Dalai Lama. I believe it is human nature to survive and the Dalai Lama makes clear how to achieve it. "Love is the absence of judgment." Quote from the Dalai Lama. Yes, judgment is human nature but we can do something about our nature. If everything is either love centered or fear centered, I try to make love my normal everyday nature. To truly love, I see no necessity to judge.

Thank you, Dalai Lama, for washing that horrible book right out of my hair. Oops, my head I meant to say.

August 29

TIME TO LAUGH

There is always time to laugh, just like there is always time for prayer. Laughter is the chili pepper of my routine, spicing up the hum drum of daily chores. It does the body a world of good and relaxes the mind. It is my belief, laughter is part of recovery. My first meeting was punctuated by laughter before it started. I had not a good laugh in a long time before I made it into the rooms of AA. I had some hearty laughs from the first meeting. I had a good laugh in today's meeting and all the 9000 meetings I have attended inbetween. In my writing and in my speech, I try to highlight the funny side of serious topics.

My rule is to laugh with you and not laugh at you. I use my own experience for a good laugh. I have enough joke material in my own life to do a comedy stand-up routine. I have broken my sarcastic tendencies because it hurts people and is not really humor. The word sarcasm means tearing flesh. Humor using a sexist or racist theme misses the mark especially in these sensitive times. Laughter works well to break tension and has an equality factor when all parties laugh together. All of my meaningful relationships have laughter as a key element of the loving chemistry.

My sponsor always referred to Rule 62, "Don't take yourself so seriously." When I work with others, I try to make them laugh as part of our communication. It establishes a heart-to-heart relationship instead of a head-to-head one.

August 30

THE PACE OF NATURE

"Adopt the pace of nature, her secret is patience." Quote from Ralph Waldo Emerson. Nature has so many messages for us. I have become a student anxious to pick up the hints God has given us in our environment. All living creatures have unique methods of survival. Someone wrote, "Even a mouse does not rely on one hole for escape." I know there are many doors open in my life and if one closes God has opened a window somewhere. I need to be patient enough to find it.

The tide taught me the ebb and flow of energy. Sometimes I am perplexed and can't seem to get anything done. Then the tide changes and bursts of energy allow me to complete meaningful tasks. I just need to accept the pace of my own personal tide. This COVID-19 has forced the whole world into patience. Some are fighting the reality of the virus. It will pass at its own pace. It is a test of patience for each one of us. I have used the time to learn new things, improve my diet, my exercise and my work.

It took many years for me to hit an emotional and spiritual bottom. It stands to reason it will take many years to kill off the beast I created. The good news is, God granted me lots of time to do the job. He is patient with me.

August 31

SECRETS

Part of my life was spent behind the black curtain. We were called "spooks" by the rest of the normal world. In movies this kind of world is portrayed as exciting, romantic and exotic. I can tell you from direct experience it is none of those things. It is dirty, nasty, back stabbing stuff. Secret agencies get their power from knowing something nobody else knows. If they share it, they lose their power. The result is Pearl Harbor and 9/11. I signed so many fear documents that said if I even dream about the secrets I was allowed to know about, I could be eliminated with extreme prejudice.

Those days are over but I still wonder if I am completely off the hook. Sort of like the Mafia, when you get old and retire the Mafia doesn't let you wander around the olive garden un-attended. For us in recovery, secrets can be fatal. We need to drop the curtain and expose all our secrets to the light of day. All. So many of us have taken our dark secrets to the grave. My spiritual teachers tell me God will forgive the worst pos-sible behavior. God knows, you know. The final step is to say it out loud to another human being. Doing so brings describable freedom.

Thai people love secrets. If you tell them to keep a secret, rest assured it will be on the street faster than electricity. It is hard work for the brain to have a secret compartment. Rigorous honesty has no secrets.

September 1

A REASON FOR LIVING

When I sat alone in my room drinking all day, I saw no reason to keep on living. I placed myself under house arrest, afraid to go anywhere for fear of a DWI. I didn't answer the phone. Afraid to pick up the mail. I saw no reason to communicate with another living soul. My career was finished. I had no new job even though I was broke. I had no more goals or dreams to fulfill. Lonely, broke, sick, depressed, I had not one reason to continue living. I had one obligation pushing me into treatment. If I balked, I would be dead now. I did meet the one obligation. It saved my life.

I did not have the desire to stop drinking. The group greeting me for the first AA meeting gave me a reason to come back. They assigned me as the literature person. I wanted to hear the next speaker also. Then each step had a reason behind the action. I felt better. I had a reason to stay sober for one more day. Each day gave me a reason to try for one more until I got to my inventory. Cleaning up my past was a good reason to continue. Repairing the damage was yet another worthwhile reason. Finally, I was able to help others, a giant reason for living.

The leap from no reason to thousands of reasons for living has been a wonderful transformation. A new meaningful, purposeful life today. A do over. If I ran away 27 years ago, I would have missed the joy, happiness and redemption.

September 2

WHERE IS THE LOVE?

If you are expecting love to come to you, then you are in for a long wait. Many of the guys I sponsored were hungry for love even though they didn't have much sober time. I understood how they felt because I went over the same bumpy road. I told them you can't expect anybody to love you when you have low self-esteem. You need to love yourself first before anybody can really love you. My first meeting, they told me they would love me until I loved myself. Truer words were never spoken. Love comes from your own heart not from outside forces.

I also explain, during the first year, huge changes are happening. You are a work in progress, especially in the beginning. Much work on inventory and amends are required to become a whole person instead a jig saw puzzle of loose parts. How do you expect somebody to love you when you don't know who you really are? Love is not selfish. Alcoholics have a selfish center. It takes time to reach a balance and think of others. It took years to get myself ready for love.

"The thing for you to do, then, is fill your own heart with Love, by thinking it, feeling it, and expressing it; and when this sense of Love is vivid enough it will heal you and solve your problems, and it will enable you to heal others too. That is the Law of Being and none of us can change it." Quote from Emmet Fox *Around the Year,* page 244.

MISUSE OF RESOURCES

God has blessed us all with personal resources which we can utilize for our lives. He gave us choices, intelligence, judgment and the power to reason. Looking back, I could see all my problems came from the misuse of my God given resources. I spent family monies on booze and my selfish pleasures. Money better spent on the kids' education and their needs. I stole time from my family and my employer to practice my alcoholic adventures. I kept my intelligence and judgment in a fog, not functioning to the benefit of anybody. I was wasting all the resources available to me. I was totally self-centered.

In recovery, I have been able to turn my will and my life over to the care of God. I have become more open-minded, less self-centered and grateful for the resources God has granted me. By relying on God's guidance and strength I have been able to learn how to use the tools I have been given. Recovery has given me a design for living which includes the proper use of resources. These resources are to be used in helping others instead of selfish pursuits. Giving instead of taking and wasting. Finally, I am able to use my intelligence for good purposes. The fog has cleared.

God has provided me with the blueprint, the tools and the power. The rest is up to me. I will be spending the rest of my life making living amends for all the resources I have misused over the years.

September 4

TODAY'S SPEAKER IS GOD

Of the more than 9000 AA meetings I attended, a good percentage were speaker meetings. The secretary introduces Tom, Dick or Harry as today's speaker but really God is speaking. Since God is working through other people the speaker has a Higher Power. He is sharing his experience in a language I can understand. Over the years I have collected some gems of truth now woven into the fabric of my recovery. Even if I don't like Harry, his message may be just what I need to hear. Not everything said sounds like God. If I listen closely, His words come through to me.

I have been on a spiritual path for many years. I ask my Higher Power to direct my thoughts and the words I write and speak. My prayer is for my experience, strength and hope to be helpful to others. My meditations I write all are a product of prayer, meditation and some research. It is a labor of love to express the spiritual lessons I learned as one alcoholic to another. When I have a chance to speak, others may find something useful and discard my poor attempt at humor. At least they know I speak from the heart and care about recovery.

I came to believe God is in every one of us. Reading the bible just doesn't work for me. I like listening to a speaker full of gratitude and love pour out his or her heartfelt message of hope. Then I know I heard from God.

September 5

WHAT GOD EXPECTS

We talk a lot about expectations and our problems associated with unfulfilled expectations. What about God's expectations of us? I never thought about it. Emmet Fox has some good thoughts on the subject, "So you have a divine right to expect all these good things from God. But what does God expect of us? Well, God has a right to expect that we will put Him first in our thoughts. Then God expects us to have a lively faith." Quote from Emmet Fox *Around the Year*, page 246. We know the best way to demonstrate our faith is through prayer. God is always listening. He hears our devotion and questions.

In my daily prayer I make a number of promises to my Higher Power. The time line is for the next 24 hours and I renew those promises again the next day in prayer. First, I promise to stay sober and do a number of things to ensure I stay sober. I certainly would not want to break my promises to my loving Father. He has kept all of His promises and never failed to answer my prayers. My promises are small really, just improve a tiny bit today. Just do the next right thing. Not project too far into the future is my 24-hour focus.

God does not expect me to perform beyond my capabilities and limitations. God is first in my thoughts and actions. If I fall short of His expectations, I will try harder tomorrow.

September 6

THE DARKROOM

"Fear is the darkroom in which all of our negatives are developed." Quote from *A New Day*, page 258. Fear is indeed a darkness in our minds. One negative thought leads to still another, spreading like a virus invading our thoughts. We lose our peace and serenity and replace it with our worst-case fears. We lose our compass and become adrift in the darkness of our own personal darkroom. I have seen fellow members go so far as deep depression and finally suicide. Permanent darkness. Positive thinking removes the need for a darkroom in the first place.

One of my spiritual teachers says, "Glance at the negatives but focus on the positives." In a real darkroom, once you open the door to light, all the negatives are wiped out. If you seek the One who has all Light the result will work the same way. Shedding light on your negatives will show some were just an illusion and the real ones need to be accepted. A strong faith reassures us whatever happens is suppose to happen. Prayer will strengthen your faith, especially in troubled times. Your Higher Power will not forsake you. He will lead you out of the darkness.

Our egos are fertile breeding grounds for our fears. We are afraid of losing something we desire or something we have. If we give our fears a reality check most will go up in smoke. We can close the darkroom and walk away.

KINDNESS AMENDS

When I decided to do my amends, I waited way too long to get started. Much time passed and I moved many times, causing damage in every location, to say nothing of the dozen countries I practiced my disease. Some people on my list had passed and more were untraceable. I harmed people I didn't know who just happened to be around me. For example, I was at a nice restaurant with a group of my drunken buddies. There was a well-dressed couple sitting at the table next to us. They were celebrating something, quietly. Being the loudest most obnoxious member of my group, the couple gave me a disgusted look. They left somewhat upset.

These nice people I never saw again. I have no idea where they are. I can still see their faces. I know I was wrong and upset them. I owe an amends plain and simple. How can I make an amends? My friend, the Dalai Lama helped with the joy of indirect amends. His religion is kindness he will tell you, "If you adopt kindness in your heart and soul it will show." Every person who crosses your path will see a smile, hear an encouraging word or two. I hope I cross enough paths with loving kindness to equal the people I have offended by my alcoholic antics.

Every day of my new life is an adventure in living indirect amends. I am now aware of the character defects which caused the need to do the amends. I try not to add to my amends list and pay my old debts.

September 8

A LIVING COMA

One job I had after leaving the military taught me some valuable lessons. I worked in the State of Hawaii Department of Corrections for three years. It was human warehousing for a number of years for crimes committed. I was an inspector, making sure the inmates had proper water temperatures and enough lighting, etc. When I entered a cell, the lights would be off most of the time. The inmates were not sleeping. They were just doing time in the dark. I asked them what they thought about. They all said, "Nothing." One smart inmate told me, "If you stop thinking long enough it is like a living coma."

I never forgot the concept of a living coma. I compared it to my thought process when I was drinking. My brain was constantly telling me things I didn't want to hear. I just wanted my thought machine to shut up and quit making me feel guilty. Solution, drink until the brain quits talking. Just like the prison inmate said, I was in a living coma not producing any meaningful thoughts. This coma led to no action because no ideas were in play. I went years without really exercising my God given intelligence. I read nothing, wrote nothing and didn't say much either. My body was in a living coma also. My only exercise was bending my elbow.

Thanks to the grace of God, I am now awake from my living coma. I will continue to use all my faculties to the best of my ability.

Facing Criticism

It has been many years since I felt the need to criticize anyone. I have enough things to correct in my own inventory without getting into someone else's sandbox. The problem is you are judging when you criticize. You think you know better or you are a better person. Sponsoring other alcoholics gives you some skills in suggesting instead of criticizing. Alcoholics are sensitive and don't like to be criticized. I know I don't. It is better to give an example from my own experience. Let the other person connect the dots without sticking a knife in his ribs.

What about when someone criticizes me? How do I face it? I remember when I was just learning to be a pilot and one instructor told me, "You don't fly very well." Absolutely worthless statement. I got a real instructor who told me why I didn't fly well and how I needed to change. Constructive criticism works for me. It does not have to be hurtful and nasty. Loving guidance instead of condescending language is best. When someone feels the need to criticize me, I chew it and swallow it. What other people think of me, is none of my business.

Being in service for alcoholics will test your tolerance. If you bring cookies to a meeting, someone will tell you what is wrong with your recipe. Alcoholics are great critics. It's so much easier than action. Service for AA will teach you how to face criticism head on.

September 10

DESTRUCTION VS. CONSTRUCTION

In my past, I have been in both the business of destruction and also construction. Sort of positive and negative pursuits. In the destruction phase of my life, my goal was freedom by bombing the hell out the opposition. If a supply truck was headed south on a trail, I would destroy the truck. If I wasn't destroying something, I was planning destruction. I can tell you for certain, none of the destruction I was part of accomplished a damn thing. Nada, zip. In Laos I filled in one of my bomb holes as a token gesture but there are thousands more. Destruction did not bring peace or freedom. It just made a mess.

In sobriety, I had a job with a construction company in Hawaii. They had noble principles and safety was their number one priority. When I drive in Honolulu, I can say I had a part in the construction of H-3 Highway joining the south side of Oahu island with the north side. I had a part in the construction of a one-of-a-kind tunnel cutting through one mile of volcanic rock. These projects will last for decades to facilitate travel. Much more productive than dropping bombs, plus nobody shot at me during construction.

This is the story of my life, the destruction phase was when I drinking and destroying everything in my path, causing wreckage for me to clean up. When I finally made it to the construction phase in recovery, I was able to build a new life from the ground up. I had to clean up my mess first.

September 11

THE THIEF OF TIME

"Procrastination is the thief of time." Quote from Edward Young. When I was drinking my entire life was procrastination. I put everything off because to do most things you need to be sober. Seeing the dentist, renewing your driver's license, going to the bank, showing up for work all required being sober. I preferred to drink rather than get something accomplished. Everything was fear based in my drinking days. Procrastination is 100% fear. Fear of being found out, fear of failure, doing nothing appears to be the only option. It snowballs into broken promises, health issues ignored and relationships' problems.

There is no good side to procrastination because you know action is required. The weight of unfinished business gets heavy on the brain. Procrastination destroys any chance of serenity. One of the benefits of recovery is the concept of action right now. I was taught, "Do it now, for I shall not come this way again." Eliminating procrastination from your character defects list has all sorts of benefits. It gives you more time, the most precious of all gifts. It improves your relationships because you are more dependable, more available.

I try to not let uncertainty hold me back from action. We never have total information. Maybe some risk is involved by acting quickly. I ask my Higher Power to help me minimize the risks and give me energy for prompt action.

September 12

THE ART OF CONCENTRATION

My mind has no clutch and my thoughts wander without purpose. I had to learn thought control from scratch. Growing up I only concentrated on the things I enjoyed. I would get high marks in history class and flunk mathematics. In order to graduate I had to focus my concentration on math and pass a makeup class. Surprisingly, I learned to like math and took advanced courses all the way to differential equations. I know if I put my mind to something specific, I can achieve my goal. I do have control over my thought-life.

In my new life on the road to recovery, I can improve my concentration skills into an art form. My daily goal is to learn new ideas and seek truth. I know my spiritual life is important. I concentrate on spiritual growth and all the aspects of God's will for me. I have to tell my body to be still. Otherwise, I play with my phone, put something in my mouth or distract my concentration in bodily stuff. I shut off noise makers like the TV or the computer. Then I move my mind through a predetermined path. I enjoy my mental journeys immensely.

It is not straining my brain. It is relaxing to sharpen my thought-life for good motives. I have a keen interest in learning spiritual truth. Right action will be sure to follow. The more I concentrate the better I get at it.

September 13

WHY WAIT FOR TROUBLE?

My daily routine is trouble prevention by solid prayer and meditation in close contact with my Higher Power. There is a very old saying, "An ounce of prevention is worth a pound of cure." True both in the material world and the spiritual realm. Are you the type person who waits until your tooth hurts before you will go to the dentist? You may be the kind of person who waits until you are in trouble before you call on God for help? It is good you do enlist the help of your Higher Power in times of need but why wait for trouble? I like to be out in front when difficulties arise instead of being in a state of panic.

In my first hour, I have a conference with my best friend, my Higher Power. He has all the power and I have none. Through our partnership there is nothing we cannot handle together. Alone, I am screwed when my fat is in the fire. I used to be the other type person, calling on God in emergencies only. He came through every time. Today, I don't wait around for trouble. It will come sure enough but I am at the ready line. God is no longer just a pinch hitter. He is the One who's will I seek constantly. He will guide me out of my difficulties. I try to do the best things for my body, mind and spirit ahead of time.

My line of communication with my Higher Power is open always. I don't need a red phone or a panic button to push. He is right here, right now.

September 14

THE BEAUTY OF SLEEP

Sleep can be difficult if your life is fear based as mine was for more than fifty years. When your mind is spinning, rest is not good. Your body suffers the consequences. If your waking hours are in turmoil your sleeping hours won't be much better. I know when I was drinking, the alcohol would make me pass out. That is not really restful, healing sleep. Resentments, dishonesty and dangerous surroundings all rob one's sleep. It is common sense we need quality sleep to function well when we are awake. Sleep is not a luxury, it's a requirement. My body needs to heal.

Before the 1950s, most people believed sleep was a passive activity during which the body and brain were dormant. "But it turns out that sleep is a period during which the brain is engaged in a number of activities necessary to life—which are closely linked to *quality* of life," says sleep expert Mark Wu, MD. I give my brain spiritual topics to feed my brain while I sleep. My subconscious is working away while I rest. Nothing wasted. There are stages of sleep from wake to light sleep to deep sleep and rapid eye movement where dreams occur. My favorite. My dreams are fantastic and I remember them.

Being in recovery taught me the beauty of sleep. With no resentments, no chaos I sleep with the angels.

September 15

ARE YOU DYNAMIC?

Being dynamic sounds like an admirable character asset. When I was on the Air Force speaker circuit, I was introduced as "a dynamic speaker". To be honest I was loud, aggressive and forceful. I had some good motives but I also had an overblown ego. Here is a better definition of dynamic, "A dynamic person is one who really makes a difference in the world; who does something that changes things or people." Quote from Emmet Fox *Around the Year*, page 267. By this definition Mother Teresa, Gandhi and the Dalai Lama come to mind. All humble, spiritual people who helped others as a way of life. All three have taught me spiritual truths.

My spiritual teacher says the secret to a dynamic personality is to believe God works through you and put His service first. If you are sincere and practical in your efforts you will be dynamic. None of us need to be world beaters or gurus. We can change our life and have a dynamic recovery program by the definitions above. If I am to help others it would be good for the newcomer to view me as "dynamic". My sponsor changed my world for the better. He was sincere and honest. I hope I have done the same for those I sponsor.

When I think about our AA fellowship, we can say it is dynamic. It has made a difference in the world. It has changed millions of people who were hopeless drunks into useful members of society. No heroes, no fame just results.

September 16

IT'S NOT COMPLICATED

"In character, in manners, in style, in all things, the supreme excellence is simplicity." Quote from Henry Wadsworth Longfellow. If we really learn to stay in the now, life is not complicated, just one moment in time. We like to think ourselves to be complex, complicated beings. This is an egotistical exaggeration. None of are so important to be labeled complicated. Just because our brains are muddled with too many inputs and an undisciplined thought-life. A better word would be confused. If we disregard our human limitations and over-extend our capabilities, the complication is our own doing. We can simplify life by changing our priorities and our attitude.

Let's get simple. When you wake up are you alive? Yes, OK great start. Now for us alcoholics we need to do some simple steps to stay sober today. All the rest you turn over to your Higher Power. Simple. Do the next right thing for 24 hours and start again tomorrow. I have found spiritual pursuits simplify. Material pursuits complicate. All my problems I thought to be complicated had a simple solution. Ask God for help. Complication is more a state of mind than reality. I seek simplicity as a way of life. I want to be free of baggage, worry and anxiety.

Simplicity is on my gratitude list. I have learned the value of changing my complicated way of problem solving. Love is not complicated.

September 17

KILLER GOSSIP

"Fire and sword are but slow engines of destruction in comparison with the babbler." Quote from Sir Richard Steele. Some folks engage in gossip as a form of entertainment. The first problem with gossip is we have incomplete information. Most assuredly we do not have all the facts. Participating in gossip indicates you think you are better than the person you are talking about. You are trying to elevate yourself by belittling your victim. It gets worse, now you have elected yourself judge. You pass out your brand of judgment and maybe even punishment. As a bonus, your story gets passed on incorrectly with new twists as the gossip takes on a life of its own.

There is no good side to gossip. It is negative, harmful and hateful. Character assassination causes harm to everyone involved. Gossip invariably discloses personal, intimate information which may be true or false. It makes no difference. It is not our job to use weapons of pen or tongue. As we write or speak with poison, we are poisoning ourselves. Everybody gets sick. Even the Pope stated gossip is worse than the virus. The people you draw into your confidence to spread gossip don't fare any better.

I know many times I was the subject of gossip. The stories were laughable and creative. When I was drinking, I provided a lot of gossip material for those who enjoyed judging me. I just stopped providing opportunities.

September 18

WORK

There was an old TV show where the main character, Maynard G. Krebs, would shriek in fear when the word work was mentioned. It does have a negative element for most folks. To me, working is digging a ditch in the hot sun with a deadline. Yet we hear in recovery rooms things like, "You have to work your program," and "It works if you work it." Doing what is required to keep your sobriety and progress is not work, it is a joyful effort. You need not work up a sweat doing the steps. The steps work on your growth not the other way around.

In recovery you are just now doing the things you should have been doing all along. When walking a spiritual path, the word work just doesn't apply. Is prayer work? It is my method of communicating with my Higher Power. Is helping others work? I sure hope not. It is an activity that helps keep me sober. It makes me feel like I am doing the right thing. I prefer to look at my spiritual activities as a loving enterprise in growth. I have dropped the word work from my vocabulary.

My point is to stay in the positive thinking mode. I try to make all my actions a joyful experience. There is nothing painful about my daily routine. Work is something I did years ago. I didn't like it. I quit and retired.

September 19

SURRENDER? LET ME COUNT THE WAYS

I was properly mangled when I crawled into the rooms of AA totally defeated. I knew I was at a turning point. In my insanity, I could only expect a down turn even further south. My first meeting I heard, "I do not have to fight anybody or anything anymore." An option I never thought of before. I had no concept of surrender. I had to surrender to the fact I needed help. I could not pull myself out my tailspin on my own. I had to surrender to a Higher Power which was a foreign idea. I had to surrender to the fact my past religious education gave me no tools to begin a program of recovery.

The key that opened the door wide for me was, surrender is not punishment, it is love. I had no idea what real love was until the fellowship embraced me with unconditional love and assistance. I found surrender to be a way of life. I surrender every day and look for more areas I need to let go of. Really, surrender is just another word for acceptance. I accept reality as it is today, not as I would have it. I had a rock too heavy to carry. My past. I finally dropped the rock and started all over again.

We are truly blessed to have the chance to live two entirely different lives. My past life is dead so I might do the right stuff this time around.

September 20

THOUGHT PATTERNS

Our thought patterns are programmed from birth and are developed through learning, education and our experiences. It is a matrix, broken into compartments for: relationships, job skills, athletics, hobbies and all different aspects of life. The matrix is limited by: lack of knowledge, funds, social status and finally by our self-imposed limitations. Our thought patterns remain inside this matrix. The boxes inside our matrix expand or shrink. Negative thinking and fears tend to shrink our thought patterns and the boxes inside our personal matrix. Alcohol accelerates the shrinkage.

In my matrix, I mistakenly thought, my thought patterns could handle: family, job, my drinking, and other relationships. I had one big box in the middle with a bottle of booze. This was the center piece of my thought patterns and my main focus. The nearby boxes like family and job lost their priority. Limitations began shrinking my matrix. No growth or expansion of my thought patterns were possible. At my bottom, the booze box was the only one left. It was shrinking like a noose around my neck. My thought patterns told me I had no way out.

Today, through the power of prayer, positive thinking and sobriety, I can stretch my matrix. I can remove most of my self-imposed limitations. I can add boxes to the matrix and expand my horizons. I can think out of the box.

UNFULFILLED POTENTIAL

"There is no heavier burden than an unfulfilled potential." Quote from Charles Schulz. I was plagued with guilt growing up because my mother harped on me not living up to my potential. It did my heart good when I saw the *Peanuts* cartoon with Lucy putting the same guilt trip on Charlie Brown. I tried to fulfill my parent's expectations but always fell short. This added to my low self-esteem. I gave up trying to do better than my capability. Finally, my parents gave up on pushing me. It was a heavy burden for so long I gave myself a vacation and began backsliding and drinking.

With no more goals, I lost my drive and failed to use my God given talents to progress. What little potential I had was extinguished by my alcoholism. Along the way I had opportunities to fulfill my potential. I refused to grow. I thought I was in teacher mode instead of learning mode. Soon what I had to teach was ancient history anyway. When I got into recovery, it was clear all my talents and potential were on hold for decades. Today, I am open to keep using the potential God blessed me with.

I can define my own potential and not worry about the expectations of others. I may never reach my full 100% potential but I am moving in the right direction. I stretch my limits every day.

September 22

ATTITUDE TOWARD CHANGE

Resistance to change is just part of human nature. I know when my routine gets interrupted by a new rule or some annoying obstacle to doing things my way, I don't like it. If somebody attempts to change me, I fight back. When I think about it, putting down my last drink and never picking up another one for decades is a monster change. One of my favorite speakers in AA always says, "I've changed." I have also heard in the rooms, "You don't have to change much, just everything." I need to change the person who drank into one who will not drink again.

A great cartoon just came out showing a caterpillar and a butterfly sitting at a table having tea. The caterpillar says, "You've changed." The butterfly says, "We're supposed to." I need to change character defects hindering me from helping others. I need to change my attitude about change. I need to embrace change where it will improve my life, improve my relationships and open new horizons. I have certain things I do which work well for me. Maybe there is even a better way if I can open my mind to change.

When you get older everything begins to turn to stone and you lose your flexibility. All the more reason to shake up your habits and daily routine. I want to be a butterfly today. I know what it is like to be worm. I've changed.

September 23

Relapse Prevention

I have done workshops on slip prevention in the past. I dusted off my worksheets. None of us, me included, is shielded against a relapse. Slip is too nice a word if the person does not make it back. I have seen too many of my fellow alcoholics die from a slip. The relapse has started way before the drink. The majority of people say, "I quit going to meetings." Pulling away from the safety of the group makes you vulnerable. The next item I hear about is resentments. We know the number one killer is the poison of resentment. Alarm bells should ring loud and clear as soon as resentments begin.

After a period of sobriety when life is going well, we tend to get over confident. We get comfortable and forget the danger. Then we slack off our principles which got us sober in the first place. Every slip is a product of negative thinking. We can feel negativity creeping into our thought-life and put the brakes on. Don't get: Hungry, Angry, Lonely and Tired. HALT. Those four usually come in bunches. EGO, Edging God Out, is another warning. Depression is a deep darkness hard to combat also.

My point is relapses don't just happen. It takes some time to cook up the poison brew before you actually pick up. It doesn't matter how many years of sobriety you have. A drink is an arm's length away.

HERE COMES THE BALL

The ball is in the air coming right to you. What are you going to do? Catch the ball? You don't have to catch the ball. You have a choice, let it drop on the ground or catch it. In my life, I thought I had to catch every ball I could reach. The concept of letting it drop just wasn't in my character. I had to learn to make good decisions on which balls to catch and which to let bounce away. My natural tendency was to catch every ball. I had to learn a new word. No.

My bosses over the years knew I would accept every project thrown my way. I was always under stress trying to please those above me. Now I can pass on a project. Even in AA, I don't volunteer for every chairmanship. I let others have a chance to be in service. At one time I was doing five different roles for my group. Finally, I let the ball just bounce off the floor. I always described myself as pro-active. I had to learn some balance. "No, not this time boss. I have a trip planned with the family."

Not catching the ball is new behavior for me. Now I embrace it. When the phone rings and I am doing something else I let it ring. I'm not on call anymore.

September 25

THE BOND OF MUTUAL ADVERSITY

Down deep in each one of us is the desire to help our brothers in peril. I have seen a special bonding in combat which comes from survival instinct. The most satisfying missions were those where we could rescue a man behind enemy lines. There is something about adversity that draws people together in a special bond. I have a combat friend of 50 years who traveled thousands of miles to comfort me in a time of grief. We are survivors of many life and death situations. We are loving brothers forever.

Is this disease not a life-or-death situation? This is no difference than combat. Most of us flirted with death before we grabbed onto the life preserver. Like souls sponsored us, helped us and encouraged us into long term sobriety. This special friendship is forged in steel, based on a common cause to stay sober and help others achieve sobriety. I know I must treat my disease daily. I have a host of friends I see every day in meetings to stand guard. Somebody has my back 24/7 so I know I am not alone, ever.

It is a sad fact some of us have to die in order for us to remain vigilant and be grateful for the precious gift of sobriety. I have seen enough loss of life to remind me what happens if I trip and fall.

September 26

SPIRITUAL EXPERIENCE

A spiritual experience need not be a burning bush. The two times I was sure to lose my life I prayed to God for help. In both cases an unusual chain of events happened. I performed some unusual actions to help myself. Two extraordinary men saved my life by chance in both scenarios. I believe it was God's answer to my prayers. When I survived both events, I had a spiritual experience. Nothing mattered but the fact I was alive. I couldn't pack a suitcase to leave the country. I was grateful to the grace of God for sparing me. In recovery, on my tenth day sober, I suddenly realized I lost the compulsion to drink. A blessing, a miracle and a spiritual experience.

I continue to have spiritual experiences as a result of doing the steps on a daily basis. The 12th Step promises a spiritual awakening. I can testify this was true for me. Meetings can produce spiritual experiences also. I heard an old-timer discuss firing a Higher Power for a new one. I followed the advice and it changed my life. I heard in a meeting we change so much in recovery a relationship from drinking days may not work in sobriety. True for me and helped me go through a divorce with love. Every day of life is a spiritual experience as I pray, meditate and seek God's will for me. It is a process not just one event.

My spiritual experiences have changed me and changed my life for the better. What I have gained from these experiences are part of my actions in love and service to others.

LESSONS FROM MOTHER TERESA

Mother Teresa is one of those dynamic persons who have changed the world we live in. Many of her famous quotes are about love. Even though she passed away 23 years ago, her spirit lives in many of us. In my collection of notes for my morning meditation I have one I will share, "The fruit of silence is prayer. The fruit of prayer is faith. The fruit of faith is love. The fruit of love is service. The fruit of service is peace." Quote from Mother Teresa. This is in direct harmony with our AA program. Another quote, "There are no great things, only small things with great love."

This next one is a daily goal of mine, "Spread love everywhere you go. Let no one ever come to you without leaving happier." To go along with this wonderful message is her constant reference to a smile. "Let us always meet each other with a smile, for the smile is the beginning of love." And this, "We shall never know all the good that a simple smile can do." A lot of what this Catholic nun says is close to what the Dalai Lama says. I try to tap into the spiritual wisdom of these great teachers. In my morning meditation, I feel like I am having coffee with my friends, Mother Teresa and Dalai Lama. All three of us are smiling.

All of us in recovery are so blessed to have found a love-based way of life to replace the fearful days of the past. It can all start with a smile.

September 28

PROMISES, PROMISES

Lately I have been writing about all the promises found in the *Big Book*. For every one I have found I can give concrete examples of those promises coming true. I know this design for living really works. I can pass on the program to others with confidence. But what about personal promises? We hear great intentions but the way to hell is paved with good intentions, as the saying goes. We cannot build a reputation on our intentions and promises. Only through actual performance and solid action can others see our true nature. "Don't tell me, show me," is the mark of real progress.

For me, it is better to not promise anything I am not sure I can deliver. Today I remain in between the white lines of my limitations. It boils down to being reliable. Setting a good example by actions not flowery verbiage. In the business of sponsoring others, it is very important to "Do what I do," by attending meetings and being in service. Being reliable went out the window when I was drinking. I had work emergencies all the time, which was code for being at Happy Hour. The sad part was I was OK with being unreliable.

Happily, today if I make a promise, I live up to it. Other folks can rely on me to do what I say. I try to let my actions demonstrate my character.

September 29

GROW OR DIE

Nature has messages for us if we listen and learn. A plant has two options, one is to continue growing the other is to die. God takes care of the garden with rain and sunshine out in the forest where no humans live. The plant in your house requires your attention and care to continue growing. If the plant is ignored it dies. The same with our recovery program. It needs our daily love and care to continue growing. Our program should have life, just like the plant, it is a living organism. If our program dies, we become vulnerable to die also. I have witnessed many deaths just like I describe.

Once life gets better, we tend to slack off watering our program. Less meetings, less service and less contact with our Higher Power. Your program doesn't just dry up and blow away at first. It is insidious and slow to decay but the trend is going in the wrong direction. I tell the guys I work with, as your sober time increases, you need to nurture the program more not less. Growth in recovery comes in the last three steps. These are growth steps not maintenance steps. If your program comes to a standstill you are going backwards, like it or not.

Your recovery will have a long life and will grow in proportion to the care and feeding you give it. Putting it on hold doesn't work. I see old-timers quit doing what got them to be old-timers. Growth or death.

September 30

GOD'S LIFE PRESERVER

When I review my past on decision making, I can see why I was such a lost soul. First, I never consulted my Higher Power to help me. Second, I hardly ever consulted someone else's opinion in my decisions. After all, I knew best. Third my motives were always selfish. No wonder I ended up on the wrong path. In my military career, God threw me a life preserver three times and I refused it. I could have had a nice quiet, normal family life with my wife and children. My ego couldn't handle normal. I had to go for the dangerous stuff to shoot for the cover of *Time* magazine. My ego almost killed me.

When faced with a decision and you pick the wrong way, maybe you will learn a valuable lesson. If you pick the right way you are lucky. Some of my wrong turns ended up to be a blessing later on. Today decision making is a breeze. I pray, ask my Higher Power for help. I talk to other alcoholics. I carefully examine my motives. Completely opposite of the old way. Now I can trust my intuition in decisions and go against conventional wisdom. I no longer evade making a decision through fear.

The most important decision of my life was to put down the drink. All the following decisions were much better when I acquired a Higher Power and made love based decisions. Today I think of others when making a decision.

October 1

GOOD FEAR, BAD FEAR

"God planted fear in the soul as truly He planted hope or courage. It is a kind of bell or gong which rings the mind into quick life and avoidance on the approach of danger. It is the soul's signal for rallying." Quote from Henry Ward Beecher. My spiritual teacher says, "Man's greatest enemy is fear. If you really get rid of fear concerning danger it has no power to hurt you." We can never be totally fearless. Today we can get help from our Higher Power to deal with fear. Before we stood alone shaking in our boots. Now we have plenty of help from God, prayer and the fellowship.

If we are doing the next right thing, we have done our best. The rest is up to God. Let the chips fall and accept life as it really is not as we desire. The question they ask big important people is, "What keeps you up at night?" To which there is a reply with a list of fears that bother leaders and politicians. Ask me the same question. I will say, "Nothing at all. I sleep with the angels."

There are so many opportunities for fear in the outside world. You need not sign up for a dose of uncertainty and unfounded fear. Fear knocked, I answered and no one was there.

October 2

FROM A SMALL SPARK

Many spiritual leaders use fire to describe the enormity of God. The simile is used to show the relationship of God and man. We are a small spark from the main source which is God. Since we are of the image and likeness of God, we have the same qualities as the main fire. Our individual flames are of the same nature and potential as the parent flame. We can ignite other flames in the same manner also. It reminds me of how our program works passing on the message of hope.

I had no spark at all until I accepted defeat and chose recovery. It started small and has grown over the years, although flickering at times. One drink and my flame is extinguished. My Higher Power has led me out of the darkness of my past. He is my partner to keep my flame burning right now. "Thou wilt light my candle, the Lord my God will enlighten my darkness." (Psalm 18:28) My job today is to set the bright example for others to benefit from my flame.

In various Buddhist functions I have attended it is an honor to be chosen to light the candles to begin the ceremony. In most religions, candles are symbols of God's grace. I am grateful to have enlightenment for a strong bright flame today.

October 3

CHARACTER BUILDING

The sum total of our actions, words and accomplishments adds up to a character profile. A legacy if you will. Before I finally decided to change my life by putting down the drink, I was proud of my legacy. When I did my inventory, I realized all my character assets were actually defects. The legacy I was about to leave this world with was one of broken promises, broken relationships and broken whiskey bottles. It was a spiritual moment when the garbage guys at 5 a.m. hollered out, "Somebody had a big party last night." They were making reference to my trash can full of bottles and beer cans.

I was up fixing myself a drink in time to hear the garbage collector announce my true legacy. There was no party. I was all alone producing garbage and nothing else. In recovery I made a decision to trash my old legacy and develop an entirely new character. I needed to build a different personality from the ground up. This time around it would be built on spiritual principles instead of money, power and prestige. I am so grateful to God for giving me many years to change my character and leave a legacy of love.

All the horrible events that led to my bottom turned out to be the best things to ever happen. A sarcastic garbage man sent chills down my spine and began a new look at reality. I should find him and thank him.

October 4

DRIVING OUT YOUR REAR-VIEW MIRROR

One of my favorite Grandma stories is about the time Grandma had to scrape some ice off her car in order to drive to church. She did a great job of cleaning the rear-view window and a poor job of cleaning off the windshield. We asked Grandma why she did such a good job in the back to which she replied, "I want to see where I have been." We all cracked up laughing. Later I thought about how much of my own life was driving out the rear-view mirror. It is so much clearer looking backwards. Of course, the real problem is the road ahead. All the lessons of life are on the road behind me. I know I need to focus on the now. I often forget to clean my windshield properly.

I tried to hang on to my past and tell stories from my archives. Soon the audience was tired of adventures from ancient history. Nobody was particularly interested in living my past with me. The past is real events whereas the future is unknown. It is much easier to hang your hat on the stories of yesteryear. They can be useful to help others "Been there. Done that." I have real empathy for the still suffering alcoholic. I try to curb my war stories and focus on improving the present so the future will be on track.

What I see out my rear-view mirror is clear only to me. No one else can relate totally. I pray I may pick parts of my past helpful to others.

October 5

OH GOD

Upon awakening in the old days, I used to say, "Oh God. I have a headache. I need a drink. I have a mess at work. I don't want to get out of bed." Notice my pattern. I called God's name but didn't ask for help. Then it was I, I, I. Every day was painful and self-centered. An awakening with negativity daily for years at a time. Today upon awakening I still say, "Oh God. Thank you for another day of life. Thank you for another chance to do some good. Sponsees with questions to answer. Many good things are in store for today." Big difference. Positive, thankful, happy, energetic and thinking of others.

Today every awakening is a spiritual awakening. Gratitude is in the first thoughts of the day. Looking for God's will for my next 24 hours with joy and enthusiasm. No chores or drudgery on the day's horizon, only good thoughts and good actions. Then I connect with my Higher Power, my partner. My prayer time is a time of enjoyment. I say the same prayers but they hit different cords each day. The first hour is my best hour because it is positive, encouraging and energy producing.

I am where I want to be, with who I want to be with and doing the right things. Nothing is missing from the picture. This is the good life. Oh God, thank You.

October 6

BRANDING YOUR DIFFICULTIES

Out on the range the cattle farmer brands his livestock with a special marking. If one of his cows stray from the herd it will be returned to him. Emmet Fox uses this example of branding to illustrate how we attach ourselves to things we need to get rid of. Plus, the things we claim as ours. Once we brand something, we form a mental connection or bond. For example, if you say, "my arthritis" you put your own personal brand on arthritis. You really want to be relieved of this malady. You don't want to embrace and hold it close. Treat the arthritis as a stray and send it off.

When it comes to resentments, we brand an adversary. "Bill is my enemy." Then you connect yourself to Bill in your thoughts. Bill belongs to you. He might as well move in with you when actually you wish he would move to the Arctic. It works both ways of course. If you really want something put your name on it by branding it and it will be yours. I often say, "My Higher Power as I understand Him." I truly want to have my Higher Power inside my body, mind and spirit. It is our duty to claim all good things.

This spiritual law requires we make our claim, we also claim the same thing for others. I claim a loving existence and I wish the same for you.

October 7

I HEAR VOICES

We all have voices in our heads. Some we listen to and some we ignore. I hear my own voice as the main one. I have the conflict of the devil on one shoulder and an angel on the other shoulder both yelling at me. The devil always wanted to have a drink. The angel got drowned out. You can guess which voice I followed. If you drink into oblivion you might get all those voices to shut up. It only works for a while. Then the voices are really loud and painful during a hangover.

Today I can choose what voices to listen to. I try to find wiser souls than me so I may learn and grow. When I attend an AA meeting, I usually find a nugget or two from one of my brothers or sisters. The first voice of the day is always my own in prayer and thanks to God. In my first hour I hear the teachings from my readings and prayer. My meditation time is when I hear my intuition talking about the 24 hours ahead. It is a small voice so I need to have quiet and listen carefully. Some of the leftovers from the day before often become crystal clear in the morning. This is my favorite time of day. Enlightenment. Gratitude.

You often hear, "Listen to the voice of reason." I give my heart a voice. It does much better than my brain.

October 8

BALANCING THE BOOKS

The accountant has to balance the books each day before he goes home. If the debits and credits don't equal there is a mistake somewhere needing correction. This is like our daily inventory which requires balancing to close the book on the past 24 hours. The parts of the day which went wrong often throw the process out of balance. The negative needs to be corrected but not at the expense of the positives. It is just as important to examine what went well and why. We tend to focus on problems rather than solutions.

Many things in our life require balance. I have to balance my selfishness. Selfish enough to put my sobriety first and unselfish enough to help others. If I only concentrate on my character defects, I am selling myself short. I have some God given assets to be used in a good way to balance my character. I have to believe in myself in order to be a productive worker and a useful member of my community. My entire day needs balance. If I did all unpleasant chores and had no fun time, I would become miserable and depressed.

My daily plan includes a mix of positive and negative. I try to start and end with a positive note. At day's end I present myself to my Higher Power, the good and the bad.

October 9

THE EYES HAVE IT

When two people meet from different cultures and have no common language, the eyes are the best means of communication. I remember meeting a general from another country who had limited English. He looked into my eyes for a long time before he smiled. He shook my hand as if he had known me a long time. His advisor told me I passed the first test. The general thought I was of good character. A bond of trust was the result of what the general saw in my eyes. I have learned eye contact can speak volumes.

At my bottom I couldn't look myself in the eye, let alone anyone else. I noticed the folks in the fellowship had clear, honest eyes. I looked for acceptance and answers when I first got sober. When I looked other members in the eye, I got understanding and the love I was seeking. The eyes had it. "The eyes are the window to the soul." Quote from William Shakespeare. Your eyes can be kind or they can convey anger. Whatever is in your heart and mind will travel to your eyes no matter what your words might be.

There was a time when my eyes said, "I need help." Now I pray my eyes say, "I can help you." Keeping eye contact was the main point I taught my new teachers. Look the world in the eye.

PROMPTLY

Step 10 is the only Step that mentions time in any way, "...and when we were wrong promptly admitted it." How prompt is prompt enough? It is largely a matter of judgment. Actually, our whole program could have the word promptly applied throughout. I was taught to do the steps as quickly as possible. The urgency is to get the job done without long pauses or procrastination. Doing one step a year is not recommended. Then again doing the steps too quickly without prayer and preparation is no good either. Everybody has their own pace. I recommend as soon as possible.

Acting promptly has many benefits and not just in recovery issues. For example, one of my best bosses taught me a lesson in promptness. He assigned me as a program chairman of a monthly meeting which included many duties like setting up dinner and getting a speaker. The next morning, no matter how early I came to work, there would be a handwritten thank you note in the middle of my desk. He took the time to personally write a meaningful note on his official stationery. Those notes meant the world to me. I tried to follow his fine example in my actions as a result. Gratitude wanes over time.

I know I am only passing by this way once. I need to do all I can before the road comes to an end. When you get old like me you need to do stuff before you forget about it.

October 11

THE WALLS OF EGO

As a recovering egomaniac, I am aware of the dangers of an inflated ego. On one side, the wall of ego, is an overestimate of our capabilities. On the other side, is the underestimation of your liabilities. Until you learn to breach these walls you are trapped by your own ego. It can take you so far from reality you become lost in your distorted self-image. Everyone around you can see your true character as your actions betray your ego. There was a time in my history I was surrounded by powerful people. I made the mistake of thinking I was one of them.

Being just another bozo on the bus is the real me today. My self-evaluation exposed the real person I am. There are no more false walls surrounding me to be breached. My defects and my assets are clear, honest and the real deal. My ego can take off into the wild blue yonder when I am around my fighter pilot buddies. A massive ego is a requirement with my war comrades. I just don't let my ego take flight anymore. I'm grounded in every sense of the word. I was just a pawn with wings until alcohol took away my sky.

My recovery program has provided me with ego reduction in depth. Freedom is just being me without smoke and mirrors to paint a false portrait.

October 12

PRAYER IS NOT A PAIN

If you view prayer as a task, my spiritual teacher says, prayer will not work under those conditions. Some folks are told to pray. They do it like an order. Their heart is not in their prayers. This just doesn't work or bring results. Prayer is not meant to be mental drudgery or painful. Too long a session of prayer says you doubt the love of God. It means you think a great effort is required to move Him. A short prayer from the heart works much better.

Growing up, I viewed prayer as punishment. I was given ten Our Fathers to say for my sins. Those prayers were meaningless as I rattled them off so I wouldn't be sucked into hell. Emmet Fox has twenty pages written describing the completeness of the Lord's Prayer. He describes the beauty of each word. I have a new appreciation for the Lord's Prayer. It is short. I can attest, as faith increases, so does the power of prayer. The joy of prayer just gets better over time. I look forward to my time I set aside each day for prayer. It has changed me where I needed change.

Prayer is a private, personal activity different for everybody. I pray quietly for the amount of time which seems right for me. I love my prayer time because it works wonders.

October 13

SELF-RESTRAINT

When I was young, I could hardly wait to have all the restraints lifted off my shoulders. I craved freedom. I wanted to make a prison break from my jailers, like mom, teachers, and church. I made three leaps over the wall. The first to the seminary to be a priest. They returned me back to my cell. The second was to join the Marines. I was underage and got caught as I was stepping on the bus to boot camp. The third escape finally worked, I joined the Air Force at a legal age. Being unfamiliar with freedom I went to horrible extremes. I could drink with wild abandon. I lived the next few decades without ever considering self-restraint. I didn't handle the gift of self-determination well.

Then came recovery and all the talk about inventory and character defects. I heard loud and clear, "Practice restraint of pen and tongue." My inventory showed me I needed a complete overhaul in restraint. I learned to pause and consult my Higher Power before I opened my mouth or wrote a nasty note. I need not comment at every opportunity. Keeping my trap shut is a great option. All my freedoms need to be filtered for selfishness. I try not to lash out with my tongue and hurt others. I put the brakes on my aggressive, proactive behavior and thought of others. I needed to restrain myself before somebody else did.

Life proceeds at God's speed, not mine. I can testify, old age will slow you down.

October 14

PEOPLE OF PRIVILEGE

All of us came from a legacy of misfortune but our defeat became our greatest victory. Think back to your bottom and compare your life today. We are indeed people of privilege. We have a special advantage when it comes to dealing with alcoholism. We are privileged to be part of a special group to deal with our mutual disease. We have a program working for millions. We are privileged to serve our fellow alcoholics just as they have helped us find recovery. We are privileged to be responsible to be there for anyone who reaches out for help.

To maintain this privilege, we shun the limelight and remain anonymous. There are millions of alcoholics who will never find their way to recovery. They may never understand there is a way out and die earlier than necessary. We the privileged, need to set the example of sobriety so other alcoholics are attracted to our program. We may be the only version of the Big Book anyone sees. Any other special group I have been a member of had limits such as age and skill. This privilege is for the long haul. A lifetime.

We have a comradeship in a class by itself, more powerful than societies of men have ever known. I am eternally grateful for joining people of privilege in Alcoholics Anonymous.

October 15

OVERCOME YOUR DISABILITIES

Sometimes our greatest weakness can result in a victory. For example, H. G. Wells had to leave a low paying job due to poor health. His disability led him to write some great books. Thomas Edison was stone deaf and he was able to concentrate on his inventions because of his disability. The point is, whatever our disability might be, it can be a challenge to find a strength in a different area. All of us have been thrown off our usual routine by this worldwide virus. It has given me extra time to work on projects needing attention.

"To him that overcomeith will I give to eat of the tree of life." (Revelations 2:7) Problems or disabilities are part of life. How we handle them can bring us closer to God. During this coronavirus, many folks have acted out in anger and self-ishness adding to the problem. Those of us following the rules are reaping the benefits of good health. Personally, my hearing loss has been a special challenge to finding new ways to com-municate. I can still see, write and read. I have to work around my disability.

Alcoholism is recognized in many circles as a disability. For us in recovery, we have arrested the effects and placed ourselves on a spiritual path. No greater victory.

October 16

I PRAY FOR MYSELF

Is it selfish to pray for oneself? My spiritual teacher says it is the opposite of selfishness. Often misunderstood, there is a line from the *Big Book,* page 86, "We consider our plans for the day. Before we begin, we ask God to direct our thinking, especially asking it be divorced from self-pity, dishonest or self-seeking motives." My spiritual teacher says, you must pray for yourself constantly. I know not to pray for material gain like winning a million-dollar lottery. I do need to ask for help improving my character. My first thoughts are prayers for several friends of mine in serious condition. I pray for them, but I need to remember I am sick also. I need to put on my own oxygen mask before I can help somebody else.

The only way I can breathe is through prayer and connecting with my Higher Power. I need strength. I need to tap into Him who is much stronger. I love my prayer time and it does many things. The only way I can breathe is through prayer and connecting with my Higher Power. It humbles me by admitting my many faults. It sets goals: writing a friendly letter, extending my hand to a stranger, encouraging another, giving every living creature I meet a smile. My prayers set my ego aside long enough to be honest with myself. I know prayer changes me. I need to keep changing and growing. If I am through learning, I am through.

My goal is to depart from the material world and enter into the spiritual world 100%. The only method to make the transition is through prayer.

October 17

YOUR PIECE OF THE JIGSAW

All of us have a fingerprint no one else has. There is no one exactly like us. Think of yourself as a unique piece of a giant jigsaw puzzle with uneven sides, odd shaped tabs and slots. We are not part of the mosaic until we find the right fit on all sides. Then we become part of the whole picture. Until then we are just loose pieces off to the side waiting to discover our proper place. Try this location over here. No fit. Try this relationship over there. No fit. Try this job here. No fit. Try this addiction or two here. No fit. Go back in the box while other pieces find the match all around and have finished the hunt for their place.

I like to think of us alcoholics as loose pieces of a puzzle. It is impossible to find the proper place in the beautiful big picture until we find a Higher Power in recovery. No location, job or relationship will be the right fit until we become clean and sober. In my own life after countless locations in several different countries, I found my final destination. Of all the jobs I have tried in my life, I found the right one at last. My job is to help others. All my relationships fit like a glove. I fit on all sides. I can honestly say I am part of the whole.

Thanks to the grace of God, I found my place through the process of doing the 12 Steps of Alcoholics Anonymous. No longer am I a misfit. The wandering and wondering are finished.

October 18

REST

"It cannot be your duty to do anything you do not have time to do." Quote from Emmet Fox. In the past I used to feel guilty for taking a rest. There were times in the military we worked 12-hour shifts, six days a week. We were like zombies in slow motion by the end of our work day. Working longer and harder has a point of diminishing returns. Productivity is lost and mistakes increase. A high percentage of accidents are caused by fatigue. Airlines have strict rules on crew time to prevent accidents. Your body will tell you when you need to take a break.

No more do I feel guilt for taking a rest to recharge my batteries. I know myself and my energy levels vary depending on the whole system. Body, mind and spirit. If any one of the three is in poor repair I shut down. Sometimes my spirit and mind are in the go mode but my body says no. To get things accomplished correctly my entire being needs to be in harmony. I am fortunate not to have a job with a boss expecting face time and results when I require some rest. Even God rested on the seventh day according to the Bible.

We get tired when we give to others without nourishing ourselves. I owe it to myself and others to know my energy levels. If I break down sick, I am no good to anyone.

October 19

TAKE TIME TO BE FRIENDLY

This is a line in one of my prayers I say every morning. "Take time to be friendly. It is the road to happiness." When I was growing up, I was the shy one who had difficulty making friends. I was friendly inside craving friendship but afraid to open myself up to the outside world. Fear of rejection trumped the benefits of bonding. Alcohol broke down fear and lowered my fence enough to let others enter my yard. My life in the military forced me into quick friendships in order to survive. Those bonds were always short termed. Consequently, friendship tended to be shallow and alcohol centered. It doesn't take long to realize bar friends are not real friends unless you are buying the drinks.

It wasn't until my recovery began, I learned the true meaning of friendship without strings. Now I have so many real friends it is hard to keep in contact with all of them. If I can maintain an open heart it will show on my face and it makes me approachable. My actions speak louder than my smile when I extend my hand and start a conversation with a stranger. I had guys complain to me they attended a meeting and no one spoke to them. I always ask, "Did you go shake hands with any of them?" The answer is, "No."

My friends are a joy I do not take for granted. Friends are on my gratitude list. A good friend knows all about you and loves you anyway.

October 20

LEARNING TO TRUST

Trust is in bold letters on my gratitude list. Trust connects to faith, love and a dozen other items on my list. First, I trust God brought me this far and will not drop me on my head. I trust everything happening in my life is supposed to happen. Trust gives me peace of mind and a positive attitude. The lack of trust makes life fear driven and negative. I trust my family and friends. They have my back when the chips are down. Help is always available. I trust all my relationships.

I trust God's plan for me even though I can only see what is front of me. His plan works. I just need to keep the faith. Today I can trust myself. You could lock me in a room full of booze for a year. I would not touch a drop. I have developed intuition I trust and believe. My heart knows what is right. All I have to do is let my heart have a voice. I try to do the next right thing no matter who is watching.

I trust this program of recovery with my life and every-body associated with our fellowship. They have earned my trust and taught me to be a trusted servant. Trust is love.

PERSPECTIVE

During this extended lock down, I have to admit my perspective has become too narrow. I see little outside my sandbox. I know I should look beyond the horizon to the greater picture. The world seems to have shrunk. The world has not changed. I need to look at the true perspective. All of us are suffering from a loss of mobility and maybe we all need to take a trip. Since we can't travel, how about this? "There is no frigate like a book." Quote from Emily Dickinson. I would love to sail away for a new outlook above and beyond. A good book does the job.

Today I walked down to the deserted beach overlooking the Gulf of Thailand. I enjoyed the cool breeze and blue sky after a night of heavy rain. The only vessel out in the gulf was a long oil tanker slowly heading out to oceans away. I thought what it would be like in the engine room, hot and sweaty. No Starbucks, no McDonald's, just a tiny cabin for months at a time. I went back to my condo grateful for my surroundings. My confined space didn't seem so bad after all. I just needed to put my perspective back to where it belonged.

Communicating with nature is my best cure for a narrow perspective. I can see God's art work everywhere and it restores my gratitude.

THE DARK AGES

"Nothing much grows in the dark," says one of our readings. Most of us have a period in our lives we can title, The Dark Ages. For me it was October 1962 during the Cuban Missile Crisis. I was a 22-year-old airman, huddled up in what was called the "mole hole". It was deep underground, built to survive a nuclear attack. I would go six days at a time without ever seeing daylight. I was on alert during the nuclear standoff protected by a bomb shelter while my family was exposed to a high-level target area. I was in the dark and witless from fear.

When I look back on that time, I did not possess a design for living I have today. Not once did I think of God. Not once did I pray or ask for help in my darkness. I had no Higher Power to call on. I was in terror, alone and afraid. I was totally powerless. I had no hope of living longer than a few more hours. If I had the spiritual tools of the program in those days, I would handle the crisis completely different. There would be light, where there was darkness. Hope, where there was despair. Faith, everything will be as God wills it to be.

Those dark ages make me so grateful for the life I have today. The spiritual path is the easier, softer way. Not only am I out of the darkness but I can help someone else who is.

October 23

HUMILITY

Humility, you either have it or you don't. You can't take a class on it or buy some. It is a result of a spiritual process. Most of us alcoholics understand the statement, "We were egomaniacs with low self-esteem." We were the best and we were scum at the same time. Once we do a complete moral inventory, we can discover the truth of who we really are. Not the worse not the best but somewhere in between. You may be introducing yourself to a new person you need to accept. Making yourself a new friend is next.

Once you accept the real you, the next part of the process, is to learn to love yourself. You learn to be right sized. You are not better than or less than your brothers and sisters. Just one grain of sand on the beach of life. Self-love may come slowly. God is Love. Connecting often and effectively with your Higher Power, the love flow has a channel to your heart. If you look in the mirror and see an honest and helpful person, humility is in your grasp. You can say, "I'm OK."

I am an alcoholic. The true description of who I am first and foremost. I announce this fact at every meeting I attend. The highest title I can achieve is trusted servant.

October 24

LIFE IS A TEST

This is an emergency broadcast. Life is a test. It is only a test. If it was real life you would be told where to go and what to do. End of broadcast. Thank God, life is not an emergency. If it was a test, I almost flunked out. I was not ready for advancement of any kind as my disease took me down a horrible path of destruction. Body, mind and spirit were all bankrupt. I came close to checking out of this life. I was leaving behind a legacy of broken relationships, broken promises and broken dreams. Through the grace of God, I got a retest.

My spiritual belief is my spirit will live on after my body ceases to function. The test is to prepare my spirit the best I can by staying on a spiritual path until the final curtain. If I view each challenge as a test, instead of a problem, it gives me a better perspective. I have a chance to succeed and rise to the occasion and grow spiritually. Life presents a series of tests and each one added to my experience so I can help others. I pass the sobriety test every day without having a cop make me blow into a balloon.

When my life got a do-over by putting down my last drink, I enlisted help for all my tests. Today I can consult my Higher Power for my tests. He has all the answers. How can I miss passing?

October 25

BEND BUT DON'T BREAK

Our code is love and tolerance. I am better at love than I am at tolerance. Everybody has a limit to their tolerance. When it is too much to take, we lash out either by words or something physical. I like to think I bend over backwards, at times, trying not to snap when my boundaries are violated. We are not doormats. I know when I snap nothing good happens. Nobody wins. I hurt myself and most likely miss my target and hurt innocent folks. I learned from my past. I let little things slide, until the buildup of little things gets to be too much and I break.

My daily 10th Step is my opportunity to handle the bending over part before hitting my break point. I review little annoyances, discomforts, fears and apprehension ahead of time. For example, I needed to make a trip to the Bangkok yesterday, which I dislike doing. I had to go to a new destination. I knew there would be long delays waiting for doctors. Knowing all this, I talked to myself about keeping my cool, acceptance, and said extra prayers. I left the house a little early. Thai driving is always full of excitement and surprises. It all worked out as well as possible. I prepared my day properly.

Thinking of our code of love and tolerance, if we really have true love of our brothers and sisters, tolerance will follow from love. On rare occasions, I still would like to slap somebody who really deserves it. With love of course.

October 26

PRAY WITH A FEATHER

In my Catholic school education, the nuns would tell us to "Pray hard." I am sure they meant well. Emmet Fox, my favorite spiritual teacher says, "Pray with a feather—not a pickax." His advice is to pray gently in a soft manner. Prayer is a loving conversation without harshness or demands. In prayer, as in many other activities, heavy effort defeats itself. Harder, longer and louder just doesn't work. I smile often during my prayers. It gives me a light tone of voice. Even silent prayer has a certain tone of an unheard voice. God hears it.

To me prayer is a joy and usually done in a quiet peaceful environment. I am talking to my Father whose greatness is beyond measure. I am in a state of humility as one of His children. Since all my prayers are of gratitude and praise there is no need to raise my voice or express wants. A short simple prayer is just as effective as an epistle. "Thank you, God," is a prayer I say several times a day.

Prayer has a great side effect of diminishing fear. My prayers are reminders of good action, compassion, and forgiveness. It sets some worthy goals for the next 24 hours. It works for me.

October 27

MAKE PEACE WITH IMPERFECTION

"The desire of perfection is the worst disease that ever afflicted the human mind." Quote from Louis de Fontanes. I thought being a neat freak was a good thing. I finally woke up to the fact it was an obsession and a strange insanity. I also made others insane by my fussing over details. I was brought up to believe all objects must be placed in a certain way, clean and polished. Nothing out of place is acceptable. An old newspaper lying on the floor is an emergency. I have to confess some of those ideas are still with me.

A quest for perfection sets the stage for failure. I was pushed for perfection until my mother gave up on me as a lost cause. I went the wrong direction. Complete perfection was not possible thus I always fell short. If your world needs to be perfect you will never find peace and serenity. I had to make peace with my imperfection and more important, the imperfection of others. Perfection is a warped judgment needing adjustment. The pursuit of perfection no longer causes me frustration.

This is not to say, stop trying to do your best. If things don't turn as expected it will be OK. Today I maintain my inner peace in an imperfect world. It's not my job to fix it.

October 28

UNITY

Our First Tradition focuses on unity as something we must have. The survival of our fellowship depends on unity. You have heard me talk about how the 12 Steps attack the selfishness we all have in common. All of a sudden, I realized Tradition One addresses our selfishness. I should be an active part of unity and not just as an observer. This means I need to set aside my own agenda and desires when comes to the goal of unity for the group. Unity is more than a buzz word. It takes positive action by all of us, be it in our home group, our family, or our work situation.

I am blessed to have a home group that focuses on unity and has many activities to pull all the diverse groups and mixed cultures together. I am also blessed with a family who travels thousands of miles to be together as often as possible for unity and love. I lived in Afghanistan for a few years and it was a study in lack of unity. The country is made up of 17 different tribes who have 400-year-old resentments with neighboring tribes. They had only one rallying point, God. Lucky to be an American in that country because we are "People of the Book". Americans get a pass. Thank you, God.

Wrapped up in the word unity is: loyalty, love, service, dedication and selflessness. Each of us are a small part of whatever grouping we associate ourselves. I pray I am doing my part for unity.

October 29

Building Walls and Bridges

When I was in Afghanistan the first thing I noticed was walls everywhere. Cities had walls, homes had walls and other mysterious activities had walls. The country had a history of being overrun by their enemies. The walls provided some defense. These physical barriers tended to translate into their personalities. Thailand, as a neighbor to Laos, has built three bridges to cross the Mekong River to join the two countries. A few years back they were enemies with a closed border. These bridges are called "Friendship Bridges". They are well used and have been mutually beneficial to both friendly countries.

We build walls or bridges by our actions. Lonely people usually have built unseen walls to block out interface with others. I know at my bottom, I built four walls around myself. I shut myself off from people who might want something from me. When I entered the world of recovery, I realized I had been building walls all my life. I learned bridge building through the concept of humility and open-mindedness. The first bridge I had to build was the forgiveness bridge. A two-way bridge that allows me to forgive and to be forgiven. If I burn down this bridge, all is lost. I have a well-traveled bridge to my Higher Power, open both ways.

I pray I have built a wall of defense against the first drink. I pray I build bridges to those needing help. I hope they see I am open for business.

October 30

SEEK TO UNDERSTAND

One line in the 11th Step Prayer is important, "To understand, than to be understood." When you are trying to help someone else, this is the key to really being helpful. In normal two-way conversation, I spend too much time forming my words to reply back to the other person. I am seeking to be understood. The point is to reverse the process and seek to understand the person I am attempting to assist. It takes some practice to quiet my mind enough to grasp the difficulty the other person is experiencing.

We have to be good listeners. Because I am hard of hearing, I may need to ask the person to repeat himself or herself to be sure I understand. I try to put myself in the other person's shoes and have empathy for his or her feelings and actions. I must place understanding the other person first. With my wife, English is her third language thus I need to have another level of understanding. Both of us work extra hard at seeking understanding since we have many differences, not only language. We have a loving relationship thus our communication works out well.

If you observe an argument in progress you will notice both sides are voicing their position. Understanding is off the table. Listening and empathy are absent. Expect poor results. Seek to understand.

October 31

SEND IN THE CLOWNS

The song "Send in the Clowns" is a sad story. In old Vaudeville when the show was going poorly the MC would shout, "Send in the clowns!" to rescue the show. A laugh can heal a lot more than a bad show. One of my daily morning prayers has a line, "Take time to laugh. It is the music of the soul." Laughter was the first thing I heard at my first AA meeting before it started. It had been a while since a laugh came out of me. I did get in some light moments during that first hour. It kept me coming back along with all the other benefits. I am attracted to others who have a good sense of humor. When I work with others a laugh relieves the tension and shortens the distance between us.

A good laugh can defuse conflict and restore peace and harmony. A hearty laugh expands my lungs and pulls all the wrinkles out of my face. I look for the light, bright side of everyday life. There is much to laugh about. Either you have a sense of humor or you don't. I believe you can cultivate laughs in your bag of tricks. Stop watching *The Walking Dead* and flip over to Chevy Chase taking his family to Wally World. I can't pull a giggle out of CNN or Fox News. Humor is on my gratitude list, you might guess.

Today I enjoy the healing qualities of laughter and it is my friend. I can dance by myself and laugh alone. I am a big joke at times so send me in coach. I am a stunt double for Bozo the Clown.

November 1

WRITE IT DOWN

Up in the family village in northern Thailand my five-year-old nephew discovered a great tool. When he is upset, he takes his notepad and writes down his anger. After he is finished, he rejoins the family with his normal happy attitude. Writing things down does many things. It gets it out of your head and in black and white for review. It acts like a relief valve to blow off steam. The stuff you write will probably get tossed in the trash but it may save a poor verbal communication or a harsh action to regret later.

I make lists of all sorts. My gratitude list of course. There seems to be magic in the process of writing it down. It re-enforces the item into my thought machine. I make a list of things to do every morning. I am surprised to check my list at day's end and most everything I put down was addressed. Our program stresses doing a moral inventory. Not in your head, not on the computer but on a piece of paper. It becomes graphic and trends become clear. Most of all, it takes strain out of your heart. Putting it on paper takes the sting out. You need it for your 5th Step anyway.

I write a lot because it is an outlet and my art. I can't sing, paint, or play an instrument. I write to help others not make all the mistakes I experienced. I read my own stuff. It's not bad.

November 2

LIFE IS NOT FAIR

Most of us have a standard of fairness hardwired into our thinking. Unfortunately, life is not fair. If life was fair the mother of my four children would have had some retirement years but cancer took her life at a young age. I can't give any of my loved ones the extra years God has granted me. It clearly is not fair. I had to surrender to the fact life never will be fair. When I voice my idea of fairness, I am making a judgment on something which isn't my call. Ultimate fairness resides in God's hands. Once I dropped my old idea about the fairness of life, I reached a new spiritual plateau.

I have faith every event has a reason, no matter what I think at the time. If I can't change it, I need to accept life as it unfolds. As the winds change, I must adjust my sails. It is liberating to realize I am not in charge and I am certainly not a judge. As a result, my losses made me stronger. If I keep my Higher Power as my partner in all my challenges, I am confident I have sought God's will for me. It does not matter how horrible the storm. I pray all my painful experiences have made me a better person to be of use to my fellows.

To the best of my ability, I try to be fair in dealing with others. I still have an expectation of fairness. I am better able to accept whatever happens and adjust in a loving manner.

November 3

BURIED TREASURE

One of my favorite Buddha stories is about the man who had a great fortune in gems. He fell asleep along the roadside and his good friend secured his fortune by sewing the gems into his robe. When the man woke up, he assumed he had been robbed and spent the remainder of his days as a beggar. All the while his fortune was right there on his person. The message is all of us have a fortune within ourselves but we might never discover it. For all of us in recovery we have found love where there was fear, hopelessness, and sickness. I still have some gems left in my robe.

I think all of us have buried treasure within ourselves. The joy of living is showing others the riches they have but don't see or understand. "Encouraging another," is in one of my daily prayers. I try to encourage on a regular basis. I have enjoyed mentoring several people and love being a father. It provided more joy than my own successes. Sponsoring is about buried treasure and illustrates my point. Inside every drunk is a useful loving person. I know where the gems are on the spiritual path. They are for all of us. I can shed some light on where to find the treasure chest.

My challenge to you is what is sewn into your robe? You may have a great painting, a gripping novel, a loving poem, some wonderful treasure within you. The only person limiting you, is you.

November 4

BEATING YOURSELF UP

All of us, who are trying to follow a spiritual life, often make the mistake of being too hard on ourselves. Self-condemnation slows us down and causes depression and inner discontent. God doesn't expect more out of us than we can do. We forget, "Progress not perfection." We are only human with limitations. Sometimes we have to step back or sideways and even fall down now and again. High standards are a good thing as long as they are realistic. Getting impatient with ourselves is foolish since we are doing our best. We won't always be up to our expectations.

"We relax, we do not struggle." I love this line. The fox condemns the trap not himself. All us run into traps on the road of life and we get caught occasionally. We suffer a setback. Blaming ourselves is just non-productive. When you need a friend, that friend should be you. Making yourself a villain is the last thing you want. Yes, it is good to try to reach goals and improve ourselves. A positive balance is better than the negativity of self-flagellation.

If I am going to keep myself as a close friend, why would I turn on myself and create an adversary? I need all the friends I can get in rough seas. I will not fight with myself anymore.

November 5

SEE THE INNOCENCE

One of our biggest challenges in life is understanding the behavior of others. They do things we don't like and even hurt
us. We pronounce them guilty in our judgment. We start a
grudge list of wrongs and plot revenge. Love and tolerance
are off the table. We are deep into negative thinking. We are
judgmental. All of this is not good to finding a solution to the
problem. No matter what the other person has done, since we
are disturbed, there is something wrong with us. We need to
see the innocence instead of focusing on guilt. We need to
think beyond the act. Think of the other person separate from
the charges of guilt.

Underneath the most annoying behavior is a frustrated plea
for compassion. This person may not know how to be loved.
Obnoxious behavior brings attention and down deep it is a cry
for love. I try to visualize my adversary at seven years old having tragedies happen growing up. The loss of a mother, a car
accident killing family members or the house burning down.
Here I am judging a particular action instead of seeing the innocence of an entire lifetime. If I have enough compassion, I can
see this person as my brother or sister.

Looking beyond behavior gets easier as your spiritual
growth increases. I want to be part of a loving world. I need to
hold up my end by living a love centered life.

November 6

SMILE ACCOUNT

You have all heard me talk about a spiritual bank account but I have new one. A Smile Account. A smile is an investment for the future. Emmet Fox inspired me on this idea. He says, "Last year's smiles are paying you dividends today. A smile is to personal contacts what oil is to machinery, and no intelligent engineer ever neglects lubrication." A smile costs you nothing but the effect is valuable. A smile relaxes a number of muscles. If smiling is your habit the effect will add up in value in your smile account. The benefits have added up from long term deposits into my smile account.

Thailand is nicknamed "The Land of Smiles". Why? After 2500 years of Buddhist teaching one of the lessons is about the things you can give to others without any resources. Top of the list is rendering a smile. Thai people just naturally smile as a way of life. Other cultures have a hard time understanding the Thai smiles. They see them as wanting something. They would be wrong. One of the reasons I live in Thailand is my smile fits right in the norm here. I sincerely love my walks around the Thai community exchanging smiles. I have plenty in my smile account to share.

A smile speaks volumes. It says, "I am a happy person. I am approachable. I am positive." It melts away suspicion, dissipates fear and anger. It brings out the best in the other person.

November 7

FIND A ROCK

I remember from my days in Hawaii not everyone saw it as Paradise. I often heard, "I need to get off this rock." It was heaven to me. Hawaii is where I got sober. I needed to find a "rock" since I spent so much of my life adrift in a dingy without a paddle or a sail. I spent 50 years on soft sand with nothing to keep me from blowing in the wind. When I got sober, I found my "Rock." I could now build a structure and a meaningful life. The solid foundation is my Higher Power. God is constant. Always was and always will be.

I live in a mansion my Higher Power built. It started with nothing but willingness on my part. My old ideas didn't work. The first three Steps poured the slab to which a house could be built. Steps 4 and 5 put up the walls. Steps 6 and 7 put in the doors. Steps 8 and 9 installed the windows to see out. Steps 10, 11, and 12 put on a roof to keep out the rain. When I started sponsoring other members, I put in a second story with more rooms. A new dimension. New improvements are always being made to my mansion. It will never be finished.

One of the oldest symbols of the human soul is one of a house or a temple. I found the solid base my soul needed. God is my Rock.

FINDING DRUNKS

One of my talents is finding drunks. During my drinking career no matter how small the town I could find other drunks like me. A tiny neon sign with only a "M" showing, I knew I found my home for the evening. M turned out to be Miller or Michelob or Milwaukee Light, no matter, my fellow drunks were in there. I would look at cellars always popular with drunks. In Honolulu there was place with no sign called the Hideaway. You parked behind a laundry for cover. I could find the real serious drunks at 6 a.m. I loved to be with alcoholics. Interesting people.

As an alcoholic in recovery, I am still talented in finding drunks. I don't need a red neon light to find the drunks I am looking for. I just look for a circle with a triangle marking the location where I will find friends, even if I just arrived in town. The only difference these drunks are sober, many of them for decades. We are like birds of a feather gathering with like goals and interests. We have only one purpose based on love and tolerance. No bar fights here. I am at home when I find these drunks. A lot more interesting when all of us are sober.

A bonus is when I find a lost soul, shaking like a leaf, just like me at my first meeting. I get a shot at auditioning for the job of sponsor. The only real worthwhile job I ever had.

GOD NEVER PUTS YOU ON HOLD

The first hour of the day with meditation and prayer is all positive and spiritual. It is the time of communication with your Higher Power. The connection can be very clear and uplifting. Then you go about your day and negative things happen. When I speak negatively or act in a bad way, my connection is broken off from my Higher Power. When I catch myself, I can stop on the spot and call on God. He does not put me on hold. He is always there like a hotline. I can re-connect immediately without delay. It also works in time of pain or confusion. It works for anything, at any time.

Once I get into anger, "Let go, let God," is out the window. It is just as if I hung up on my Higher Power. I am saying, "OK let me handle this by myself." Why turn my back on help when I need it most? Negativity can be addictive, going deep into a downward spiral. Just plain losing your sanity. Sort of like being drunk without the alcohol. When I catch myself circling the drain, I say, "Stop, drop, and pray." I reconnect, relax and turn it over to my Higher Power. I should have made the call before the stuff hit the fan.

My daily goal is to stay in the Sunlight of The Spirit. I try to keep the hotline open when shadows appear on the horizon.

November 10

THE DALAI LAMA AND I

You all have seen me quote the Dalai Lama frequently. I refer to him as my "buddy" because we have a lot in common. He is only a few years older than me, same hair line and we both smile a lot. His religion is loving kindness. When I am asked about religion, I say the same thing. I have been studying his works for over twenty years. I have absorbed enough of his teaching it has become a huge part of my spiritual thought-life. A recent quote from the Dalai Lama, "Everyone wants a joyful life." Me too.

When I met him in Hawaii over twenty years ago, I had the instant feeling he knew me. He has a great sense of humor, is playful. He laughs hard and loud. Everything he teaches about compassion, forgiveness, and love, supplements our AA program. He spends five and half hours each day in prayer, meditation and study. He started his path at age two and I got started late but at least I started. He got rescued from sure death by the CIA in 1959. I got rescued by the CIA in 1969. We are both ex-pats. But, I pray, meditate and study just a fraction of time the Dalai Lama does. I have added more time over the years.

I know his level of spirituality is a product of a lifetime of discipline. In a small way I can follow my buddy's example and keep reaching new plateaus. I want what he has.

November 11

RAINBOW FAMILY

When I was a senior in high school, I had a sophomore girl invite me to her class dance. I accepted. No big deal, except she was Mexican. Knowing my family's prejudices, I kept the date a secret. It led to more dates and a secret engagement. Soon enough they discovered the girl I was seeing regularly was Mexican. My parents went berserk and demanded I stop. I was too far into maturity to comply. My solution was to leave home, join the Air Force and come back a year later. Against angry parents, I married this beautiful lady. We drove thousands of miles away from both our families. The marriage produced four wonderful talented children. My parents did come around after some time and loved my wife and the kids.

One cousin's daughter married a black man and the marriage produced three stunningly attractive children. Another cousin's daughter married a fellow Air Force guy. He came from an Air Force family of five brothers. He is movie star handsome from a white dad and a black mom. My Thai wife and I attended the wedding. It was a multi-colored and multi-cultured affair. No one batted an eye. We have a rainbow family successfully dropping the prejudices of past generations. I am blessed to have such a family with nothing but love.

Family is on my gratitude list. My family now includes 100 Thai in-laws, nephews and nieces. Thank God, I have broken the prejudices of my parents.

November 12

ARE YOU A RUNNER?

I have been a runner all my life until recently. I was running away from life, from reality, from myself. I had low self-esteem and fear. I discovered I could really run well. It helped me escape. I was trying a getaway my entire adult life. I ran away from home many times until the Air Force gave me wings. Now I could fly away from my messes. In a rare moment of clarity, I realized no matter how far or fast I went, I was stuck with me. In the end, I wanted to run from my wreckage. But there was no place to run to.

I always stayed super busy and over committed all my life. I could hide in the turmoil. Chaos is a great cover for character defects and bad behavior. When I got sober, I did my inventory. All my running popped up very clearly. The motives for my running were never pure. I joined the military not for service and patriotism but to run away. I am tired of running. It is hard to move me these days. I have arrived at the final destination. My home group meeting is my departure lounge. The next trip will be short. Just to the temple next door in a shopping cart.

It took some practice at standing still to finally get it. My morning quiet time with my Higher Power is the opposite of running. I can hear God better when I stop running.

November 13

THIS IS NOT A REHEARSAL

During filming if one of the actors makes a mistake, you can stop and do the scene over again. Many scenes are rehearsed first before rolling the camera. Unfortunately, in life there is no rehearsal. Every scene we have a part in is the first take. It is also the last take. There is no script, you make it all up as you proceed. Your lines are all ad-lib. People enter stage right and surprise you with unscripted dialogue. This is not a rehearsal. My spiritual teacher says, "We are in this world for the purpose of learning." Since we are learning, mistakes are expected. The point is to improve at the next opportunity.

Life as a passing show. Every scene is done once and it's over. Either we learn and improve, or we let the poor performance of the past drag us down. We can dispose of past scenes and take the lessons learned with us. We prepare for the next adventure. Life is meant to be discovery and training. Every experience we have eventually will disappear into nothingness. Since entering recovery, I noticed each scene improves over time. The mistakes are fewer. I can handle those ad-lib moments much better.

Welcoming truth into our lives is the beginning of a liberating adventure. I am happy there is no rehearsal and no script. I could never remember my lines or hit the right mark anyway.

November 14

SEPARATING THE WHEAT FROM THE CHAFF

We have a lot of chaff in our lives, distractions from the real stuff of life. The best example of chaff I can think of is the static blast of news. We get it as soon as we open our computer or turn on the TV. There is a shooting somewhere, you can be assured. Will this information help me in any way? Why am I listening to something ten time zones away I have no control over? All this kind of stuff does is turn my inner dimmer switch down another notch. A steady diet of chaff can depress you. It keeps you from more important things.

The Serenity Prayer is all about separating what is meaningful and important from those things over which you have no control. The nourishing wheat from the garbage. The acid test is simple. Do I have control over the situation? If I accept the world as it really is, then I am a winner. If I can turn over to God those things impossible for me to change, I am a winner. If I am not sure I have control over a situation, I ask my Higher Power for help. Like magic, the answer comes in my morning meditation. If courage is a problem, I ask God to be my point man in times of uncertainty.

I work hard at avoiding the chaff which is part of our culture. If I don't know the details of a mass shooting, I am OK with the lack of information. I have courage and acceptance. Serenity has found me.

November 15

ONCE MORE WITH FEELING

A popular AA joke is, "The good news about getting sober is you get your feelings back. The bad news is you get your feelings back." Only an alcoholic can understand the wisdom of this joke. I remember when I was young in school plays the director would tell me, "OK Mike, now once more with feeling." When I was drinking one of my goals was to not feel anything. Emotions and feelings were the least of my problems. Alcohol would dull any feelings popping up, like guilt or shame. Years of suppressed feelings were stored up waiting for me to get sober. Then the dam broke loose.

Once I began the road to recovery, I could start to feel my emotions. I could deal with them instead of drowning them. The process of sharing in meetings did something I had never done before. Share my inner emotions, my faults, and my life with other human beings. I never tried to express those feelings. I was taught from childhood to keep them to myself. Other wiser members then could tell me more about the underlying causes of my feelings. It seems the women are much better at processing feelings and emotion than men. I do know for sure the old gals in AA taught me so much about expressing myself openly and dropping the macho tough guy act.

All of us got a second chance at life. A big do over. I am going to do life again, this time with feeling.

November 16

THE SPIRITUALITY OF PRACTICE

It is common knowledge if you want to excel at anything, long hard practice is required. One great example of diligent practice is the story of Andre Agassi. His father drove him to excellence by early and rigorous, sometimes cruel practice. Andre became very wealthy but he never found happiness. He hated tennis and was forced to hit thousands of balls against a backstop every day. He eventually became a champion. He was not happy. He hated tennis. Finally, he had a spiritual awakening as the result of giving. A lesson we know well as a part of our program.

My point being given enough practice, great heights can be achieved. But at a horrible price. The motives need to be pure for the best results and a happy life. Agassi is now self-actualized by helping underprivileged kids in the Las Vegas area. He never wanted to be a tennis super star. For us, we have a 24-hour practice plan that works wonders for millions of us alcoholics. Happy joyous and free alcoholics. "We practice these principles in all of our affairs." As a result, we are champions every day. We do our practice every day in prayer and meditation. If our motives are not selfish and self-seeking, we reap amazing rewards.

We all are winners with only one mission. We can always improve our spiritual skills with new readings, extra ways of giving, and more service. Much easier than a good backhand.

November 17

RESTRAINT OF PEN AND TONGUE

Maybe the most important thing you have to say is best swallowed and not spoken. Most of my angry emails were deleted before they were sent. Nothing can make you more lovable than restraint of pen and tongue. Keeping quiet at every opportunity can make you adorable. I have learned it is OK not to hold forth on every subject. Emails you send then delete may be gone from your screen but it is in cyberspace forever. It can be retrieved. Once you write something down it can always backfire and give you unwanted blow back.

I had a sponsee I sent an email in an attempt to get him on the right path. He made multiple copies and gave everyone in the group a copy of my email. There was nothing in there I was ashamed of. It was not intended for broadcast but privileged communication between the two of us. As we know there is never a guarantee of privilege once your words are in print. You can ask yourself if you are harming anyone. I know I have received negative letters intended to hurt. I hit the trash can for three points as soon I get the tone.

In my home group the format calls for everyone to have a chance to share. As the group has grown, I have learned to be economical with my words and brief in delivery.

November 18

INTELLIGENCE

My friend Emmet Fox says, "It is your duty to God to run your life along intelligent lines." He points out God has given us all enough intelligence. But we use very little of it. I know I put my intelligence in a coma for decades. The only smart thing I could do is remember the recipe for ice. Today I focus on body, mind and spirit to make up for the years of neglect to all three. I feed my brain with the good stuff. It takes some discipline to control my thought-life and make intelligent decisions. The first hour of prayer, readings and meditation works well to channel my thinking in the right direction. I am asking God to help me in this ongoing mind project.

A fistful of college degrees and a high IQ have nothing to do with the kind of intelligence required for doing the next right thing. I can ask myself, "Am I selecting my readings intelligently? Am I watching my diet intelligently? Am I spending my money intelligently? Am I approaching my problems intelligently?" I know my intelligence is the light of God in my soul.

The *Big Book*, page 86, has a wonderful passage on intelligence. "We ask God to direct our thinking, especially asking that it be divorced from self-pity, dishonest or self-seeking motives."

November 19

HOW CAN I SERVE YOU?

I don't talk about service too much because to me it is like talking about air. Service is part of our recovery program. When I finally made it to the rooms of AA, they put me into service from day one. I am so grateful for a lifetime of service opportunities and the benefits of service. It has reaped great rewards. My sponsor was a service junkie with positions in 10 different separate groups. He had a "service sponsor" who told him to back off. Allow the new guys an opportunity to step up to the plate. I took the lesson to heart.

I have been in all sorts of organizations and companies and I have found in any group only a small percentage of the folks get stuff done. The majority are willing to be spectators and a small percentage complain about the few who are doing the work. I learned just because I am a "get it done" guy not everyone is hardwired the same way. I have to be tolerant to those who prefer the bench to the field. There are all kinds of ways to be in service. Not all of it has to be visible.

Service is an attitude. A positive one. I ask my Higher Power, "How can I be of service?" Not just to my home group but to the community at large.

November 20

AUTHENTICITY

When the guys I sponsor look at my gratitude list, some point to authenticity as one item for explanation. Authenticity to me translates into the real deal. When I stand before you there is no make-up, no plastic surgery, no hair piece, no tattoos and no advertisements on my clothes. What you see is what you get. On the inside I seek truth. I speak the truth as best I can. My smile comes naturally as a result of being happy, joyous and free all the time. I don't pad my resume nor do I run myself down. I can look you in the eye because I am at peace with myself and my Higher Power.

Before I surrendered and admitted I was an alcoholic, I had absolutely no authenticity. I was anything but real. I wore a mask even when I was alone. I was a phony to the outside world and to myself. Selfishness was a way of life and honesty was off the table. My life was fear driven. Being found out was my biggest fear because there were cracks in my cover story. I rode my past accomplishments like a horse. The horse died underneath me. Finally, the mask got ripped off. I stood at the turning point. I had to get real or die. It took years to get a grip on reality.

It is a wonderful freedom to be just one, real person. There is no longer a need to impress anybody. The truth is, I am a sober alcoholic. Nothing more, nothing less.

HAPPINESS FOLLOWS SIMPLICITY

Everyone who knows me will describe me as a happy guy. Quite often folks ask how can I be happy all the time. I love to respond, "When I see you, I know everything is going to be alright." Or, "Your smile brings me sunshine." The real reason is the 64 items on my gratitude list makes me happy for all the gifts God has put in my basket. Too long a list to rattle off at every opportunity. But the heart of my happiness lies in simplicity. Someone wrote, "Making complicated simple is real creativity." I agree. I strive to leave the material world by subtracting my belongings to the bare essentials. No wallet, no watch, no jewelry, just the shirt on my back.

Simplicity is freedom to me. Walking with my arms swinging is best. I never owned a backpack. I threw my briefcase in the ocean 30 years ago. More importantly is the subtraction of junk in my mind. With no resentments, anger, desires, self-seeking in my thought life, I can be free to enjoy the simple things in life. A cup of coffee with an old friend is priceless. It fills my heart with happiness. Flowers in bloom, patting my local dog, just lungs full of clean air, all simple and free.

Since I am in charge of my own happiness it follows, I am charge of simplicity. I turn over the impossible and complicated to my Higher Power. I focus only on what I can control. Simple.

November 22

Damage Control or A Design for Living

If somebody came up to me at my bar stool in Honolulu and asked me, "Hey Mike do you have a design for living?" I would finish my drink and move to another bar. I would have no idea what the hell he or she was talking about. Life before was recovering from one crisis to another. I was driving through life with a bulldozer destroying relationships and everything in my path. In crisis management and in the damage control mode all the time. Lost at sea without a port in mind or in sight.

I lost my basic education on problem solving. I couldn't get sober on my own, these AA guys could. They told me to find a Higher Power. The action plan is doing the 12 Steps. The goal is: a spiritual awakening, peace, serenity, healthy relationships, love, usefulness and more. A Design for Living just like our *Big Book* clearly states. Today I have lots of goals. I can dream again. I know which port I am sailing to. If you have a couple of hours to spare, I can answer that original question, "Do you have a design for living?" Yes, I do.

As I sat with a drink in my hand and good intentions. Not one of those good thoughts added up to action. Today my life has a design for living. I have a daily plan. It happens.

November 23

MANY FREEDOMS

Most of us lost different freedoms because of our drinking. In recovery, we have a deep gratitude for all the freedoms we enjoy today. Freedom from being locked down by alcohol into solitary confinement for years. It could have been a death sentence. Now we get a daily reprieve based on our spiritual condition. One more drink and I go back to my cell, maybe to die. Freedom from self-will run riot is such a blessing when compared to the bondage of self in the past. Freedom from the heavy weight of my past makes me want to fly without wings.

When I wake up every morning the freedoms splash over me. I live oceans away from my original home, thanks to freedom to choose where I live. I was able to choose my partner, my friends and my Higher Power. I faced hundreds of choices of how to treat my body, mind and spirit. I can make responsible choices to properly care for myself and others. Every sunrise promises another adventure in living a sober life filled with love, peace and serenity. All of these freedoms are delicate and fragile. They can be lost in a heartbeat if I make a poor choice.

Today I chose to be free. I do what is necessary not to lose this precious gift. Helping someone else remove the chains and walk out of a cell is the greatest reward of all.

November 24

BREAK THE LAW

I am not advocating cheating on your taxes or speeding on the highway. I am talking about breaking laws others laid down for you and self-imposed ones. The laws you give yourself are usually fear based. The point is, fear is unfounded. In Hawaii there is an AA meeting called Black Experience. I was told it is for black people only. I was brought up to believe AA meetings were for alcoholics no matter what color, gender, or sexual orientation. So I went. It was a super meeting with all sorts of races. I made some new friends, some of whom were black. I love black people. I am happy I broke the "law."

"Know the rules well, so you can break them effectively." Quote from the Dalai Lama. I have been a rule breaker for decades. It spices up my life and gives my adrenaline a rush. When you get older, your kids become the parent and give you rules. My daughters beg me to stay out of the kitchen when we go to a Thai restaurant in the USA. I can't help myself. I bust into the kitchen and meet the one Thai cook who is the heart and soul of the place. I speak enough Thai to make a new friend. They love it, I love it and it drives my kids nuts. Fun.

Emmet Fox says, "Why not start today and repeal some of the many laws you are sure to have made for yourself." We have enough limitations without adding ones based on fear.

November 25

CAN I BRING HOPE?

Whenever I hear the topic of hope, I think about Bob Hope. During his long lifetime he made 57 trips overseas to bring hope to young troops away from home for Christmas. He gave of himself without any monetary compensation. All of us know the feeling of hopelessness. A gift of recovery is hope. I was taught, as long as there is life, there is hope. There is no such thing as a hopeless drunk. Those days of fear, resentment and negativity are gone. The vacuum is replaced by hope to fill the void. If I take care of today's challenges today, I am assured of a bright future.

Bob Hope would visit the sick and wounded away from the cameras on these trips. I had the good fortune to be on one of his trips and saw him in action spreading hope everywhere he went. Today my heart is full of hope. I can share it with those who are in a dark place. Where there is despair, I can deliver a helping of hope by example. Every time I encourage, I receive courage. It is by giving we receive. I ask myself the question every morning, "Can I bring hope?"

Every year in recovery gets better, just like the old-timers promise. Long-term hope has resulted in dreams becoming reality. My happiness surpassed my imagination. Hope is connected to everything on my gratitude list.

November 26

Unfinished Business

Our founders knew just how to put the steps in the order they are. The first seven steps are all about you. Step 8 is just a list but more importantly is about willingness to dig into unfinished business. Not until Step 9 do we interface with another human being and the outside world beyond the rooms of AA. By the time we have reached this key step, we become whole again. When I got to this point, I could see a mountain of unfinished business. A sage wrote, "If your mission is to empty the ocean with a tea cup you better get started and find a bigger cup."

I focused on Step 9 for a five-year stretch. I flew all over the globe to the places I had left wreckage. It was the best years of my recovery by far and the most rewarding. I really wanted to start a new life with principles on a spiritual path. After I did as thorough a job as I could on my amends, I could ease into Steps 11 and 12. I could declare mission complete for the first time. When the "awakening" came to me I realized I still had unfinished business. I will have unfinished business for the rest of my life. I keep using my big cup every day.

I still have some leftovers but it is manageable. The ocean is pretty much drained down to a lake. My goal is to take care of today's business now, not tomorrow.

November 27

THE SEEING EYE

For many years my vision was blurred and distorted. I was viewing my world through the bottom of a whisky glass. It was forever empty. I was always looking for the next drink. I had a narrow field of vision with blinders on all day, every day. Now my vision is programmed with faith. What I see has clarity and a sharp focus. No fuzzy images. Faith to me means everything I see is good. God put everything where it is for a reason. My job is to see it as God intended it to be seen. The eye of the beholder gives me the gift of seeing beauty others might describe as ugly.

I can control my attitude. I can control what I see and how I see it. I don't let others tell me what I must see. Our *Big Book*, the last chapter titled, *"A Vision for You"* is a perfect ending for alcoholics. "Suggestive only." "We know only a little." All poetry to my way of thinking. I ask God to direct my thinking. When I open my eyes after meditation, I can see clearly the day ahead. The goal line is clearly visible. I can see God's handiwork everywhere I travel. His fingerprints are everywhere.

I have read the following passage from the *Twenty-Four Hours A Day* book dozens of times. I just now focused on it. "I pray that I may have a seeing eye. I pray that with the eye of faith I may see God's purpose everywhere."

November 28

GO TO YOUR SECRET PLACE

In my readings I picked up on a new way of looking at meditation. The reading describes private thoughts in your conscience mind as, "The Secret Place". If you make your Higher Power your partner, there is no limit to what you can accomplish. In your secret place nobody can invade you don't let in. If you invite only your Higher Power in as a partner in your thoughts, you have formed the most powerful team possible. This union can be blissful and inspiring. These times are when I get my inspiration. This is also where I can adjust my attitude.

You know how much we talk about resentments. You are letting the person you resent reside in your head, rent free. You can get your serenity back through daily prayer and meditation in your Secret Place. You have a fortress against the outside world in your conscience. Emmet Fox writes, "Modern psychology has shown that most of our difficulties have their roots in the depth of the subconscious." Nothing is coming out of the subconscious without going through your Secret Place. There it is met with your Higher Power, and your conscious mind.

This is an entirely new way of looking at my thought-life. I really like it. I keep trying to grow spiritually by expanding my thought-life.

November 29

FOOL'S GOLD

During the Gold Rush of prospecting days fool's gold was prevalent. Emmet Fox writes, "Old timers used to say to the tenderfoot: When you think you have found gold you probably have not, but when you do find it, you will know it for certain." I get a powerful spiritual message from this. Much of my life I was chasing fool's gold. I am a sucker for glitter and attractive packaging. The luxury car, money in the bank, house on the hill all just shiny objects. Fool's gold all of it. Bombay gin, top of the line nectar of the Gods. Will calm my nerves, help me relax, make me laugh. I was really a super fool.

Just like Emmet Fox says, what you think is gold is not. I spent the better part of my life chasing "fool's gold." I thought I had life by the tail and it was the other way around. The spiritual message is, when you find it, you will know it for sure. Yes, thank you God. I have found real gold. My recovery is the real deal. AA, the fellowship, the steps, sponsorship, service, the literature, all 100% gold. I know it for sure. Today I am wealthy in love, peace and serenity. No more prospecting.

True gold for us is to be one with God in peace and harmony. We no longer need to be in bondage of passing material objects. We also know all the real gold must be passed on.

November 30

ANGELS IN YOUR LIFE

My parents named me after an angel, St. Michael. I did little to follow the spirit of my namesake during most of my life. I grew up with idea I had my own personal guardian angel to watch over me. Over the years I still believe in angels but not with white wings and a halo. More like certain people in my life were angels in disguise. They guided me down the right road at the right time. My Aunt Jerry, for example, was close to a perfect angel. She was totally unselfish. From her heart, she wrote me a letter pleading for me to do something about my drinking.

If this letter was written by anybody else than my Aunt Jerry, I would have torn it up and trashed it. I could not turn her down. Maybe she was the only person on earth I would listen to. An angel for sure. I surrendered a week later and my life was saved. In my spiritual reading here is a quote from Psalm 91, "For He shall give His angels charge over thee, to keep thee in all thy ways. They shall bear thee up in their hands, lest thou dash thy foot against a stone." A reminder of the time I was drunk, fell and hit my head on a stone in my own front yard.

Once I quit drinking, I found new angels everywhere I go. The secret is, you need to be sober to find them.

December 1

BE AN EARLY RISER

One lifetime habit paid big dividends. I recommend getting up before sunrise every morning. When I was a young student, I found getting up early to study for a test was much more productive than burning the midnight oil. My mind is freshest in the morning. You need to be sober for best results. I was always the first one to class. Later, the first one to work. It put me leaning forward rather than catching up. In the military, being early was a plus. Today, my day begins before sunrise to greet my Higher Power just as the sun lights up my surroundings. It is the quietest part of the day, no birds chirping, no dogs barking and no electronic devices on.

Once I finish my hour of prayer and meditation, the best part of my day is done. Everything else falls in line after I have my personal quiet time. I have properly prepared myself for whatever might happen during the rest of the day. Our founders stress morning meditation and it works wonders for me. I catch my brain before it has a chance to spin up to top speed with worldly concerns. My attitude is properly adjusted before anything happens. My energy is peaked at sunrise and is gone completely by sundown. I know how to best use my energy levels.

I truly enjoy each day because it starts with gratitude, love and happiness. If you feel rushed all the time and behind the power curve, try being an early riser.

December 2

WAR OF THE WILLS

As a boss most of my adult life, I was accustomed to getting my way. If one of my staff would try to impose his will over mine, he would incur my wrath. In the military, it is cut and dry who has the hammer. However, I met my match when a civilian worked for me. I could not impose my will over her or fire her. Her job description said she could type business letters but she never typed one. The war of the wills was waged. I forced her to do a letter. She mailed out a draft letter with 40 typos to Hilton Hotels. The letter blew back in my face with my boss. I lost the war in a big way.

Much of my life was frustrating trying to impose my will over those I worked with and my spouse. No wonder resentments were a way of life with my controlling attitude. What a revelation to discover I didn't need try to push my will on anybody. The only will of importance is God's will. My job is to try to follow His will. It was such hard work to make the world operate to my specifications. On the rare occasions I did get my way, the results were pathetic. One of the greatest freedoms of recovery is turning over your will. Your Higher Power knows the right way.

I tried to use my strong will to control my drinking problem. I failed miserably. Once I surrendered to God's will, life became much easier. No more war of the wills.

December 3

THE PAIN OF EXPECTATIONS

Having expectations is just plain human. We expect the sun to rise in the east every morning. So far it has. If we go on vacation, we expect to have a good time. If you take the family half way across the country to see Wally World and find out it is not open, you lose it. Crushed expectations. Most of our frustrations in life are based on unfulfilled expectations and awful surprises. We have expected outcomes. When they do not happen, problems begin. It takes some spiritual work to not have expectations. Whatever happens is supposed to happen. No matter what we think.

If you are a control freak like me, this is extremely difficult to swallow. If we can wrap our arms around acceptance, we can begin to handle unexpected outcomes. If we get ahead of God or think God doesn't know what He is doing, we are off the path. I have faith. Sometimes it is hard to bring it to mind when I get frustrated with people, places and things. I take a deep breath and reconnect with my Higher Power in times of disappointment. I try to follow the spiritual advice of wearing the world as a loose garment. Going with the flow has to be learned after a lifetime of paddling against the tide.

The pain of expectations can be relieved by our own faith. Acceptance is the answer to all my problems. No medication required for this pain, just an attitude adjustment.

December 4

LET'S THROW MONEY ON THE PROBLEM

When I was working at a treatment center in Hawaii, a black limo arrived at the front door. The chauffeur got out and opened the back door and a rag tag young drunk hit the pavement. Daddy got out and handed me a check for 50K and said, "Fix him. I will be back to pick him up." The father wanted to buy some sobriety. The young man wanted no part of what the treatment center offered. The father returned in 28 days to find out his son had jumped the fence and was blowing in the wind. The father shouted, "All the money I gave you clowns and you let him get away."

I have found money and recovery just don't mix like oil and water. You can buy your way out of jail. You can buy the finest of medical care. You can even buy companionship. But sobriety is not for sale on any market. Betty Ford can't make you sober with the fine cuisine, the spa and rose gardens. You will just be a pampered drunk. The person must have the desire regardless of wealth. In fact, most of us were broke when we finally found the rooms of recovery. I was headed for debtor's prison. Material well-being followed spirituality.

The saying, "money is the root of all evil" is a bit overboard. But there is a grain of truth in the statement. We are blessed our program is not about money. Sobriety is priceless.

339

December 5

FINDING YOUR ART

I just read an article on being super sensitive. Alcoholics are well known for being sensitive and overly so. This expert says, "To be sensitive is good, because sensitive people are aware of a thousand interesting or beautiful things where the obtuse person gets nothing." What follows the gift of sensitivity is creativity. Most of us have art within us that got scrapped while we were in our disease. There is art yet to come out of all of us. Now we are sober, it is a good time to resurrect lost art. Art is not necessarily a painting, poetry, or musical talent. It may be the thing you do well and is uniquely you. My cousin is an artist in designing antique cars.

From *Body, Mind and Spirit,* "Art is not about making a product to buy or sell. And it is not about success or failure. Art is about connecting with nature and God and joining them in their continual act of creation." We are free to express ourselves and share our creativity. Recently a good friend published a book of poetry. It made me realize I had quit writing poetry 40 years ago. I buried a part of my art. Resurrecting your art is an important missing part of you. Writing is my art in words. It is freedom, love, expression and much more.

I hope you all have found your art as I have. It lights my fire. More importantly, to show others where their art has been hidden or forgotten, is a joy not to be missed.

December 6

THE GRATEFUL HEART

"The worship most acceptable to God comes from a thankful and cheerful heart." Quote from Plutarch. My present-day spiritual teachers echo the same sentiment. For us in recovery, gratitude leads to humility and positive thinking. My gratitude list has much positive energy. It fires up my entire system into good actions. How can I not be cheerful when I review all the gifts God has bestowed on me? I could have missed all of this joy. Through the grace of God and lots of help, I pulled out of a fatal nosedive. All of my prayers today have a thankful message to my Higher Power.

This quote I used from Plutarch, a Greek philosopher, was written over 2000 years ago. Plutarch is famous for writing *Parallel Lives* where he promoted peace between the Greeks and the Romans. He showed the similarities between two warring adversaries. Dealing with resentments is an age-old problem. Our program addresses our problem areas head on. Our 11th and 12th Steps, stress prayer and meditation. The message on how to accomplish our spiritual goals has been around for centuries. My heart has been in the cheerful zone for so long it is hard to recall the times of darkness and despair.

A love-based life automatically has gratitude and happiness at the core. True partnership with my Higher Power simplifies my life. It gives me the freedom to be creative and helpful to others.

December 7

GRUMPY OLD MEN

You can be male, female, young or old and be like a grumpy old man. All can qualify with the right negative attitude. When my eyes open in the morning I am brand new, a baby, ready to learn something. My age on the calendar is not an issue. My dials go to zero, no airspeed, no altitude. Only my prayers and spiritual literature. If my mind is open to inspiration from my Higher Power, I see myself as the most uninformed person on the planet. If my old ideas are stuck in cement, I am on the way to becoming a grumpy old man. Yes, the hard fact is, I am an old man. But I need not act old or be grumpy.

To qualify as a grumpy old man, you need to complain often with anger in your voice. You need to say things like "Back in the day." Or, "These kids don't know how lucky they have it." You need to find other grumpy old men. Next, focus on all the medical problems and operations. Rehearse all your aches and pains. Be ready to show your scars. Graphics are good for grumpiness. Have some evidence on your phone to show the other grumps. After seeing the movie *Grumpy Old Men*, I told my kids to shoot me if I ever become like those guys.

Getting old is mandatory and a blessing. Having a few years' experience, I know what works for me.

December 8

FACT OR FICTION

We are hit with so much hype and garbage every day it is a chore to separate fact from fiction. Most of us have learned advertising is a lie for the most part. The internet is full of scams. The result of all the lies we encounter on a daily basis causes us to to be leery most of the time. A quote from Aldous Huxley, "Facts do not cease to exist because they are ignored." I once saw a news clip of a military spokesman saying, "We cannot confirm a B 52 has crashed today." A giant smoke plume and fire was right behind the spokesman.

In my spiritual reading, Emmet Fox refers to God as The Truth, in caps. He urges us, "To seek The Truth," as a life long journey. God, truth, love, happiness, serenity, peace and spirituality are really all one. Fear, negativity, and falsehoods are the opposites of The Truth. In our morning prayer and meditation, we can start with Truth nothing but The Truth. We can put love, serenity and peace into our conscious mind. Then we step outside where a storm of fiction is waiting. We girded our loins for the battle.

My Higher Power will help me when I ask in prayer. I start each day with much Truth and fact. I can make it through any storm for one more day.

December 9

ARTIFICIAL SOBRIETY

Artificial Intelligence is a way of life today. When you call a bank or a credit card company, you get a recorded response. It is almost impossible to talk to a human being. A man I sponsored was into artificial sobriety. Without my knowledge, he was sent to me by his boss specifically to "do the AA thing" or else lose his job. It took me a long time to figure out what was going on. When it came to the 5th Step the show was over. He kept up his act until his boss caught him play acting. A drunken fight later, my former sponsee lost his job.

At one time, I taught a graduate level course to working adults. The second night of a five-night course, I had a new face from the first night. I discovered he was a stand-in to take notes for his boss, the artificial student who signed up. I dropped his boss, who never showed up in person, from the course. The boss complained and the university backed him up. This university was all about money and nothing to do with real education. They were passing out artificial degrees for folks who could buy a degree for advancement. I quit the university with my integrity.

Imagine building a robot to stay sober for you. The robot could go to meetings for you, do the steps and sponsor other robots. What a nightmare. Thank God for our real deal. Artificial sobriety doesn't exist.

December 10

BE A GOOD HOUSEKEEPER

My living space is immaculate because it gets swept, mopped and dusted twice a day. You could eat off the floor. It gives a comforting atmosphere of order and cleanliness. With constant maintenance and vigilance, I try to apply good housekeeping to my spiritual life as well. I remember the big chunks of garbage dumped when I did the steps. What a wonderful feeling of freedom. The trick is to keep my mental house squeaky clean. This means taking care of little problems before they become big unmanageable ones.

The big hurdle for me is relationships. I need to communicate, on the spot, when something is not in harmony. Try to resolve any issues before they turn into a misunderstanding and then into a resentment. No need to be a doormat. Disagreements can be handled with love and care instead of hostility. My old way was to stew in righteous indignation for a good while and save my forgiveness for later. Better to forgive quickly and be done with the entire matter. No dust has a chance to accumulate with this positive process. Then there are some unpleasant tasks needing attention. Some of us procrastinate until it eats away at our peace and serenity. Why not do it now, clean the shelf and be done with it?

Not waiting for a little bit of dirt to turn into a job for a bulldozer is part of streamlining your life. Better to be free with blue sky ahead. Be a good housekeeper.

December 11

CONTEMPT

Contempt is such a negative word yet it marked a good portion of my life. Then I found the rooms of recovery. Today, I can truthfully say I am without contempt of any kind. My parents had the idea we were better than everybody else. My father was plagued by contempt of just about everything and everybody. I knew in my heart that was not right. I rebelled by playing soul music and dating outside my race. Contempt is judgment plain and simple. It can lead to hate and anger. There is also a fear factor in most contempt. Even worse is contempt before investigation.

All understanding comes to an abrupt halt in contempt. Love and tolerance are off the table. Walls are built, doors are closed and minds are locked down tight. I remember having contempt for Vietnamese people before I ever went to Vietnam. I got sent there and I was able to investigate up close and personal. My contempt dissipated when I learned what the Vietnamese people were really like. I found them to be intelligent, caring, resourceful and wonderful folks. I came to love them. Holding an entire race of people in contempt is insane.

Lucky for me when I was forced to go to an AA meeting, I had no concept of what AA was all about. My normal way would have been contempt prior to investigation. I was stupid enough to get it on the first try. Thank God.

December 12

HAPPY, JOYOUS AND FREE

In our morning meditation and prayer, we are seeking God's will for us. At the same time, "We are sure that God wants us to be happy, joyous and free." Quote from the *Big Book*, page 133. In the past, my periods of unhappiness lasted for years. Today only a few bad moments. Showing my gratitude by actions is a way of life. My job is managing my happiness. The 11th Step prayer states, "That where there is sadness, I may bring joy." My mind is open and willing when happy joyous and free. I feel wonderful, fulfilled and useful.

If I am in misery, I am the one who put me there. By asking God for guidance, the answers come as requested. Today my troubles are challenges. Down deep I know there is a reason for everything. My faith shores me up in times of uncertainty. Enjoying the freedom to spread joy wherever I go is heaven. Happiness and joy have a multiplier effect. It is contagious. Giving of myself in a joyful way, I get re-paid many times over. Helping beat up drunks turn into beautiful human beings is a joy not to be missed. For the first time in my life, I have joined a winning team.

Nobody is happy, joyous and free all the time. But I can get back to my normal happy state with the help of my Higher Power.

December 13

A MAKEOVER

Need a makeover? How about some new clothes, a fancy watch, new hairdo, maybe some Botox shots? All the external stuff won't change you one bit. The make-over we all need comes from the heart. It radiates outward from true change or regeneration. First, change the way you think. My thought patterns led me in the wrong direction for years. The old way did not work. I needed a new "thinker". In the old days, I never asked God for help. My process was doomed from the start. Admitting to my inner self I needed a total makeover, formed a mental ground zero. Accepting the slow pace of the steps was required.

For change to happen, I needed to be at peace with myself and everything else. I stopped fighting and went with the flow. I followed what worked so well for my fellow alcoholics. I could see the light in their eyes. The smiles on their faces. The first obstacle to my regeneration project was my ego. My ego needed reduction in depth. It became obvious my education and history of accomplishments were all meaningless. Without a spiritual center, there was only self-delusion. It is no secret the 12 Steps will change you, if you do them thoroughly and consistently.

Today I am still a work in progress. My regeneration will take the rest of my life. I can see the change in myself. My makeover is working.

December 14

THE POWER OF PRAYER

We have no power. God has all power. We can tap into His power by asking Him. Simple. Why do we keep trying to fix stuff we cannot fix? He can if we let Him. This is a Father relationship where our Father wants the best for us. He loves us more than we can imagine. All we have to do is communicate. Look at it this way, I go to my treadmill for my exercise. The treadmill it is just a hunk of junk until I turn on the power. My feet move to get the desired result of better health. Likewise, I need the power from God to get the desired result. The only way to turn on the power is by praying.

In Thailand we had 12 kids trapped in a cave for 12 days. This entire country was praying, including me, for their safety. Plus, the kids were praying themselves. It is hard to describe the difficulty of getting to the area where they were trapped. It was a two-hour trip under water which required oxygen in heavy tanks. The ordeal was successful. The kids gave prayers of gratitude as soon as they got out. Some people call this luck. I say it was prayers. I had life and death events where I prayed ferociously. I can tell you for a solid fact prayer works. Prayer is the air I breathe.

My prayers only work when my motives are pure and I do my part. Praying for material goodies doesn't work. Praying for spiritual growth works every time.

December 15

PATIENCE AND FAITH

The principal part of faith is patience. This statement from one of my readings made me ponder. Our culture is moving away from patience to more speed and instant information. The 5G world makes one's head spin. People expect answers right now. Gigs of information instantly please. Hurry hurry, worry worry. Stop the world, I want off. Emmet Fox tells us, "Don't hurry we are going to live forever somewhere. We are in eternity now so why rush." Patience was never in my tool box until recovery. "You are right where you should be." Those were the words I heard when I became impatient. How comforting to hear.

Faith for me began slowly. When the results worked well, it grew through patience. Years of negative thinking will take years of positive thinking to reverse the flow. Fox talks about prayer, "Of course, it does pay dividends, fabulous dividends, but it usually takes a little perseverance in the face of preliminary slowness." Our prayers are always answered. We just don't know when or the form it may take. My faith grows stronger with time. I hurry less, worry less. If life seems to be going too fast, I step aside. Give myself a time out. When the race started, I was a rabbit. Today I morphed into a turtle.

Faith takes you past knowledge and doubt. Swiftness does not always win the race. Spiritual awakening takes time.

December 16

DEEP AMENDS

One of my vivid memories of basic training was the drill instructor screaming at a new recruit. "I'm sorry," said the recruit. "We know you are sorry. You are one sorry sack of..." screamed the instructor. Sorry was dropped from my vocabulary. It is indeed a weak response to a harm. Amends are so rewarding. I kept doing deeper amends. The payoff is tremendous. There is no statute of limitations on amends. If you still think about it, amends are in order. Distance doesn't matter. Death does not give you a pass either. It took years and thousands of miles to do my amends. Not once did I use the word, sorry.

Here is an example of a 40 years late amends. As a 13-year-old altar boy, I supplemented my allowance from the collection basket. I would pocket a couple of dollars every Sunday. I made the amends. My amends trip to Vietnam, Laos and Thailand changed my life. It took three years. Twelve time zones are not too far in search of an amends opportunity. Death of the person requires some creativity. I suggest you find a "like person" and do something special for them. I have never been disappointed in my deep amends efforts.

Lots of love has come my way by doing amends. It is so rewarding. It makes me want to go even deeper. I seek ways to make living amends every day.

December 17

GIFT SELECTION

When you give a gift, the manner of giving and the intent is more important than the gift itself. The Dalai Lama instructs, if you send a gift via your hired help it amounts to zero. The best is a gift from love in your heart. No strings attached. Delivered by you personally. The Dalai Lama says, "While you are engaged in the practice of giving you should do so with great happiness and radiance on your face." Your gift can cost a ton of money. If your heart is not right or your motives are wrong it's a waste. You want to select the best gift possible? How about yourself?

We have this member in our group who bakes cookies every weekend for all who come to the meeting. He follows a recipe, takes time out to make and bake. He does this out of pure love. He expects nothing in return. This is a good thing because few thank him for his efforts. Some even complain about the amount of sugar. Only an alcoholic would complain about a free lunch. Service is all about giving. The ultimate gift, yourself. Suit up, show up, set up, and clean up daily. Like is says in the St. Francis Prayer, "For it is in giving that we receive."

Giving is such a joy and fun. Every day I look for a chance to give. Today I got high fives from two small kids begging in the gutter with million-dollar smiles. My gift was small compared to the dividend.

December 18

THERE IS ALWAYS ONE

If you have ever been with a group of people on tour, there is always one. He is late coming out of the hotel. He is the last person at every stop when everybody is in their seats ready to go. To make matter worse, he does not care. There is always one. In school, one bad boy would cause us all problems. The whole class suffered loss of privileges. In my AA home group, we have a group conscience everyone has a chance to share. There is always one who takes up too much time. Pointing out this breach only brings more agitation.

Having been in a lot of different groups, there is always one. Why is it a fact there will always be a pain in every group? My theory is, God wants us to learn patience, love and tolerance. God wants us to be respectful of those who are different. Some people act up in a cry for love. Negative attention is better than no attention at all. Our rule says, "If we are disturbed there is something wrong with us." God has put all sorts of people in our path. We are not going to like them all. We have an AA saying, "If you like everybody you meet in meetings, you haven't been to enough meetings."

In life it would be good to accept the fact we are not going to be happy with everyone. If we search for God in each person, we might find something we are missing.

HALT

When I was just starting my road to recovery one of the most meaningful suggestions was called HALT. Don't let yourself get hungry, angry, lonely and tired. HALT Usually, two or three of those things happen at the same time. It is a warning to stop and fix these threats to serenity and sobriety. Being cool and patient requires extra effort as expectations unravel. In recovery, we know to care for body, mind and spirit. If the body is in an unhealthy state the whole system is in danger. Temporary insanity is quite likely.

In early sobriety I took a trip from Hawaii to Boston. It was a red-eye trip. I got no sleep the day and night of the trip. I thought I could purchase a snack on the way to San Francisco. No food this particular flight I was told. No problem, only five hours to San Francisco. Hungry. Tired. After landing it was 3 a.m. and no restaurants were open. Angry. On the flight to Boston, a lady with a crying baby sat next to me while she slept. Lonely. Tired. No flight attendant in sight. Really hungry. I get up seeking food. None on this flight either. Angry. HALT

I made it to Boston without drinking but was in rough shape. I remembered HALT and said some prayers. I was temporarily insane but I didn't act on it. My recovery principles saw me through.

December 20

GET HELP WHERE YOU ARE WEAK

In grade school we were tested on verbal and math skills. Scoring high in verbal, I was low in math. At a young age I was mentally programmed to do poorly in math. I loved English class and hated algebra. One summer got ruined because I repeated geometry after scoring a "D" during regular class. Somehow my attitude got changed. Determined to beat this mental block I had about math, I found geometry fascinating. Scoring an "A" I went overboard. I became a master at math. Accepting my shortfall, I learned to seek help where needed.

Teamwork is such a wonderful thing. It has a multiplier effect of the whole being better than the parts. Having been on a few successful teams, I could see where the best skills of some made up for a lack in others. In my home group each member is good in one important activity. We don't have people in positions of authority, only trusted servants. Our society is just what we alcoholics need. Perfect for us. Strange to the outside world. Individually we are weak but as a group we are winners. There is a wrench for every nut in the room.

One promise says it all, "We will suddenly realize that God is doing for us what we could not do for ourselves." I accept my weaknesses. I look to others and my Higher Power for help.

December 21

YOU CAN'T HAVE BOTH

We have heard you can't have your cake and eat it too. Emmet Fox has a whole list of like applications in the spiritual sense. For example, "You cannot have peace of mind, and have your ailment too." The two just don't mix. Fox has many hints about ailments. Why claim ownership to your affliction? He suggests thinking of God. Turning your ailment over and putting it out of your mind. How about, "You cannot have power in prayer, and the luxury of resentment and condemnation too." We know resentments stop love and serenity like a brick wall. Our minds are going two ways on a one-way street. Guaranteed headache.

"You cannot build a new consciousness and a new body and live mentally in the dead past too." Living in the now is part of our life today. Wallowing in the past steals a part of life happening right now. Life in re-wind. "You cannot have harmony continually unfolding in your life and enjoy gossip and criticism too." Again, oil and water talking love and harmony while bad mouthing others we don't like. Dropping your complaints on the operation of the universe will set you free. Heard in the rooms, "You can't be hateful and grateful at the same time." Gratitude fills the heart with love and happiness.

My favorite is, "You can't have complete faith and be fearful at the same time." Real opposites we can apply to our daily life. The unknown belongs to my Higher Power. Faith will shelter me in any storm.

December 22

REMORSE GOES AGAINST GOD

Remorse was in my thoughts doing my Steps. These feelings of remorse are wrong thinking. If I have remorse, I am denying God's forgiveness. Remorse is not accepting God's will for us. Emmet Fox says, "Repentance does not mean grieving for past mistakes, because this is dwelling in the past, and our duty is to dwell in the present and make this moment right. Worrying over past mistakes is remorse, and remorse is a sin, for it is a refusal to accept God's forgiveness. This means that you should change your thought and know the Presence of God is where you are."

Emmet Fox has made me ponder long and hard about my thought-life. Often, I play back the old tapes of my war stories. What I really need to do is stop the tapes. This is all about behavior modification for better things right now. The big chunks came out in my 4th Step. Time to press on. Simple really. I was in this mode for so long, I did not see the way out. I need to keep reading, praying and listening to my fellows in the meetings. Emmet Fox says remorse is a "sin". I almost missed his message because I quit believing in sin a long time ago. Sin or not, I had a lot of remorse.

Remorse, guilt, and blame are all a waste of time. All things past don't help me improve today. I will have better tomorrows. I ask God's help to open up my mind, just like this passage did.

December 23

PROGRESS IS LIKE THE TIDE

Progress in recovery was not a straight line upwards. It is more like the tide with a back and forth flow of success and setbacks. If a mountain was straight up and smooth you would not be able to climb it. My mistakes, however painful, stick to my ribs more than my successes. My slips take time to heal and reflect on where I went wrong. I try to not repeat my errors. The point is to keep the upward goal in sight no matter how many times I fall. Those bad decisions are helpful as I try to help a struggling alcoholic on the same mountain.

Just like the tide, we need to be relentless in our movement. Each ebb and flow bring a new level of spiritual awakening. If I look back to where I came from, I never want to slip back down into the black pit. Keeping my bottom green is important lest the memory of all the pain fades. In nature, autumn time the trees shed all their leaves and look to be dead. But in spring the trees blossom and come back to life even stronger than before. If I stay with the flow, I get stronger. I surprise myself with new revelations and new ideas.

Not much in life seems to be in a straight line. There are bumps in the road and detours requiring some navigation. If I lose my program the downward fall will be straight to hell. Been there already. I don't want to go back.

December 24

SELECT A MOTIVE

Behind every action is motive. Doing an inventory of your motives can be revealing. There may be an array of motives. For just one act there is the motive you tell others you have. There is the motive you tell yourself. Maybe the real motive is buried in your subconscious and needs to see the light of day. It takes some thought and time to make sure you have examined all the motives. "We consider our plans for the day. Before we begin, we ask God to direct our thinking, especially asking that it be divorced from self-pity, dishonest or self-seeking motives." Quote from the *Big Book,* page 86

When people find out I live in Thailand they assume they know some of my motives and do my inventory. How wrong they are. Those folks have no idea we have strong AA here. Many motives are in play. It does not matter what others think my motives are. I know why I am here. A list of twelve honorable and good motives can be spoiled by one rotten motive in the mix. I pray for right thinking and chip away on my selfish nature. I noticed my motives take care of themselves. The action of doing the next right thing wipes out the wrong motives.

Only my Higher Power and I know my true motives for each of my actions. There may be some subconscious motives I am not really aware of. More will be revealed.

December 25

LOVING KINDNESS

When I write my offerings to all of you, I pick a topic and think about it for a couple of days. Meditation helps me to come up with some thoughts to pass on. In my spiritual readings, I came up with the topic of "loving kindness". My friend, the Dalai Lama, says his religion is kindness. I have read his writings and find they resonate with everything I believe. Compassion is a key part of loving kindness my study showed. It is a way of life I am trying to adopt. I am sweeping out some of my old ideas. I learned if I am pushed, I need not push back. This is a total new concept for me. Kindness is not pushy.

The idea of helping those less fortunate should be part of the actions you do every day. Having a good heart and good intentions is just so much smoke if it doesn't result in action. Compassion and loving kindness need to be part of your blood and bone. The culture of giving versus one of taking is why I live here in a Buddhist atmosphere. In my short meeting with the Dalai Lama, I could feel the loving kindness in person. What a wonderful warm feeling I received from this encounter. I later realized why. Loving kindness is who he is.

It would take many more years on a spiritual path to be anything like the Dalai Lama. The idea of loving kindness is stated in the St. Francis Prayer I say every morning. "It is by giving we receive. To love than be loved."

December 26

FAMILY SICKNESS

Our disease is not confined, it has spread to our entire family. Families by their very nature have problems and our alcoholism ensures our families will suffer. Every family has something the matter. We can stop some of the madness by our actions in sobriety. The chain of pain can be broken by love and tolerance at home. We can set the example of harmony. Our loved ones slowly will appreciate us again. It may take a lifetime. It is up to us to change the family's opinion. There is an old saying, "The family that prays together stays together." Did not happen as I was growing up. I had no idea what a family should be like.

It was not until I got into recovery that I developed a sense of family. My AA group became my family to start. Then I was able to begin to repair my own blood family. My son's diagnosis of ALS was a big family event which bonded us all. We gathered frequently to share what little time my son had left. It was a total love story. It brought joy out of what could have been sadness. Today I am able to be there for my family. The nice part of this story is other branches of the family have picked up on the importance of being together. Some of our gatherings have reached almost 100 relatives.

For my part, my family has long forgiven me my drunk days. They respect my sobriety and don't talk about my alcoholism. I am just another family member.

December 27

TRAIN OF THOUGHT

Having lived in various cultures I know there is a wide variety in thought processes worldwide. Eastern or Asian thinking is quite different from Western or American thinking. The term "train of thought" is probably not meant to be a metaphor. But the deep groove of thinking is like a freight train doing 65. One track, lots of speed and no deviations. I saw the two trains of Vietnamese thought collide with the train of American thought up close. My job was to advise the Vietnamese Air Force. I was on the wrong track. I immersed myself in Asian culture for the last 15 years. I now see the error of my ways.

Living in an international community for all this time now has taught me my train might be going in the wrong direction. The choice is to be flexible or be frustrated. I have adapted to the Asian-Thai culture since I live here. If I get angry at a Thai person and raise my voice, they shut down. Communication in a soft, peaceful manner is all Thai folks understand. Not to say one culture is right and the other is wrong. Let's just say, different. In my morning meditation, I ask my Higher Power for direction of thought. It does not matter what culture I happen to be in. God doesn't prefer one culture over another. We are all God's kids.

When traveling back to the USA, I suffer reverse culture shock. Security agents at the airport screaming at me rattles my cage. A smile and gentle reminder would be nicer.

December 28

WHAT YOU BLESS

Today's title centers on you becoming what you think. You become what you are by the actions you perform. Painters become painters by painting, in simple terms. In a spiritual sense, we become loving and tolerant by acting in such a manner described as loving and tolerant. The thought and action of blessing a thing is positive. The blessing will be returned to you. The easy part is to bless your close friends for their love and assistance. Most likely they will bless you back in kind. If you have enemies, bless your enemies. The power to hurt you will be dissipated. Whatever in your life you find troublesome, bless it and it will gradually fade away.

The other half of today's message is, whatever you curse, it will curse you back. When my car doesn't start, I kick the fender and curse the hunk of junk. The result is sore toes and the car still won't start. Negativity begets negativity. Pounding our fists on the steering wheel is no good for us alcoholics. God bless this traffic jam. Nothing positive will ever come from cursing. If I push an enemy, he will push back. Better to give him a hug. Bless him in your prayers.

The true and tested method of handling a resentment is to pray for the other person. Picture your adversary as a small child. Try to imagine all the tragedies of his or her life. Maybe you can bless him or her as a friend.

December 29

GUILT MANAGEMENT

One comedian said about guilt, "The gift that keeps on giving." Guilt can work to our advantage if it is managed correctly. Guilt can be a call to action instead of an anchor on your butt. Simple rule, if you can do something about the emotion you feel, correct the problem rather than procrastinate. If you are powerless over the thing you feel guilty about, put it in the forget box. Part of my self-management is not to let anyone else declare me guilty. Nobody else can make me feel guilty without my permission.

The guilt I need to be free from is the past, over which I am powerless to change. These are unfortunate events in our inventory. By now we made direct amends where possible and indirect amends where not possible. God has already forgiven us. Refusal to let go of these thoughts is refusing God's love and grace. It is important in the inventory process to get it all out. Old events do not get better with age. They must be owned and discarded. Guilt must go in the trash with blame and shame.

My guilt management is a balance between self-blame nudging me into positive action on one hand. Versus what God has already forgiven on the other hand. Unless I am in a court of law, a judgment of guilty from others is their problem.

December 30

TAKE YOUR BRAIN TO THE GYM

Let's take your thought-life to the gym. First is diet. I took the seven-day Emmet Fox mental diet last year. The results were fantastic. In my male dominated AA group, the language has always been salty. Part of my mental diet is to eliminate unnecessary words in writing and speech. The diet worked and the salty words have been deleted from my thought-life and speech. How about pushups on reading? Have you added some meaningful readings to give your brain some muscle? Get some parts of the mind working in new territory? Maybe your thinking needs a scrub.

How about some pushups on negativity? Time to review what is negative in your thoughts. Pray for a reverse flow of energy into the positive. Mend a broken relationship by breaking the ice in a positive loving message. Try a handwritten note. How about your prayers? For me, I make sure to stop and work my brain on the words. I let them walk me through the woods for a while. The same prayers have changed their meaning as I have changed. The point is our thought-life needs discipline. The best work-out is a good regimen with goals for stretching knowledge and understanding.

You don't need a sweat band or Gatorade in the brain gym. But you might feel physically tired. We really only use a small part of our brain anyway. Our learning has no glass ceiling. There is plenty of room up there.

December 31

HEART VERSUS MIND

"The mind cannot long act the role of the heart." Quote from Duc de La Rochefoucauld. Thankfully, I was taught to give my heart a voice before I open my mouth. My heart knows what my mind has yet to comprehend. Here in Thailand, they have 750 terms for the heart. A person's character is described by the type of heart the person displays. No matter what you say or the look on your face, your true heart shows through. My mind can try to cover up what is in my heart. It will not work for long. My heart is good and my mind is defective. I have learned to filter what is in my mind through my heart before I speak or act.

My mind is like a boiling tea pot. My heart is quiet and moves slowly. My morning meditation and prayer is all about listening to my heart before my mind gets up to a boil. My intuition works only when it is quiet and peaceful. I fill my heart with gratitude which leads to love and happiness. When I was drunk the connection between my mind and my heart was broken. My mind was dictating action and thought with poor results. Only in sobriety does anything meaningful come from my heart and mind. By years of working a spiritual life, I changed who I am.

"We must combine a good brain with a good heart." Quote from the Dalai Lama. I work on improving my brain. But I give my heart the last word.

MORNING PRAYERS

I PROMISE MYSELF

Today I pray:

To promise myself to be so strong that nothing can disturb my peace of mind.

To talk health, happiness, and prosperity to every person I meet.

To make all my friends feel that there is something in them.

To look at the sunny side of everything and make my optimism come true.

To think only of the best, to work only for the best, and expect only the best.

To be just as enthusiastic about the success of others as I am about my own.

To forget the mistakes of the past and press on to the greater achievements of the future.

To wear a cheerful countenance at all times and give every living creature I meet a smile.

To give so much time to the improvement of myself that I have no time to criticize others.

To be too large for worry, too noble for anger, too strong for fear, and too happy to permit the presence of trouble.

CHANGES

Today I pray that I may understand there are some things I cannot change:

I cannot change the weather.

I cannot change the tick of the clock.

I cannot change another person against their will.

I cannot change what is right and wrong.

I cannot change the fact that a relationship ended.

I can stop worrying over that which I cannot change and enjoy living more!

I can place those things into the hands of the One Who is bigger than I.

Save energy. Let go.

Instead of trying to change someone else:

I can change my attitude.

I can change my list of priorities.

I can change my bad habits into good ones.

I can move from a place of brokenness
    into wholeness, into the beautiful
        person God created me to become.

TAKE TIME

Today I pray that I can:
Take time to think.
>It is the source of power.

Take time to play.
>It is the secret of perpetual youth.

Take time to read.
>It is the fountain of wisdom.

Take time to pray.
>It is the greatest Power on earth.

Take time to be friendly.
>It is the road to happiness.

Take time to laugh.
>It is the music of the soul.

Take time to give.
>It is too short a day to be selfish.

Take time to work.
>It is the price of success.

Take time to do charity.
>It is the key to Heaven.

LIFE IS A CELEBRATION

Lord, help me today to:
Mend a quarrel.
Seek out a forgotten friend.
Dismiss suspicion and replace it with trust.
Write a friendly letter.
Share a treasure.
Give a soft answer.
Encourage another.
Manifest my loyalty in word and deed.
Keep a promise.
Find the time.
Forego a grudge.
Forgive an enemy.
Listen.
Acknowledge any wrongdoing.
Try to understand.
Examine my demands on others.
Think of someone else first.
Be kind.
Be gentle.
Laugh a little.
Smile more.
Be happy.
Show my gratitude.
Welcome a stranger.
Speak your love.
Speak it again.
Live it again.
LIFE IS A CELEBRATION!

THIRD STEP PRAYER

God I offer myself to Thee to build with me and do with me as thou wilt. Relieve me of the bondage of self, that I may better do thy will. Take away my difficulties, that victory over them may bear witness to those I would help of Thy power, Thy love, and Thy way of life. May I do Thy will always.

Amen

Big Book, page 63

SEVENTH STEP PRAYER

My Creator, I am now willing that you should have all of me, good and bad. I pray that you now remove from me every single defect of character which stands in the way of my usefulness to you and my fellows. Grant me strength, as I go out from here, to do your bidding.

Amen

Big Book, page 76

ST. FRANCIS PRAYER

ELEVENTH STEP PRAYER

Lord, make me a channel of Thy peace
> that where there is hatred, I may bring love
> that where there is wrong, I may bring the spirit of forgiveness
> that where there is discord, I may bring harmony
> that where there is error, I may bring truth
> that where there is doubt, I may bring faith
> that where there is despair, I may bring hope
> that where there are shadows, I may bring light
> that where there is sadness, I may bring joy.

Lord, grant that I may seek rather to comfort, than to be comforted
> to understand, than to be understood
> to love, than to be loved.

For it is by giving that we receive,
> it is by forgiving that one is forgiven.
>> It is by dying that one awakens to Eternal life.

Amen

Twelve Steps and Twelve Traditions, page 99

Made in the USA
Middletown, DE
27 May 2022

65736650R00212